October 2005
Shape / Men's Fi
Cru

YIN YANG FITNESS

The Whole Package of Health

壽

Dear Elizabeth:

what can we say about our very special friendship forged over juvenile food sculptures, bawdy stories and "naughty Laurean" lectures? (that was oddly specific...). We must stay in touch and find ways to visit or work together. Our families seem to mesh so well. It is an honor to call you a friend.

Love, Kent and Maria

AMBERWOOD PRESS

www.amberwoodpress.com

Kent@mylifefitness.com

ISBN: 0-9726026-0-7

The Yin Yang Fitness program is intended for healthy individuals age 18 and over. This book is solely for infomation and educational purposes and is not medical advice. Before starting the Yin Yang Fitness program or any other exercise program, you should consult your physician. We suggest taking this book to your physician and any other alternative health practitioner you see regularly. Let them see the exercises to be sure this program is safe for you.

Amberwood Press
P.O. Box 3814
Ventura, California 93006-3814
On the web: www.amberwoodpress.com

Cover photography by Jeff Douglas
Cover design by Sandy Douglas
Make-up by Jodi Malitsky
Weight training photography by Zach Johnson

Printed in the United States of America
Printing by Advance Color Graphics, Buena Park, California
10 9 8 7 6 5 4 3 2 1

This book is dedicated to our parents—four people who gave us the love, time, patience and freedom to pursue our dreams with confidence.

THANKS...

We would like to thank Jeanne Kalogridis, a dear friend with enormous talent who gave us the confidence to undertake this project in spite of the odds; Karin Fraki, MS, CSCS for her friendship, expertise and belief in us; Rich, Kim, Mark and Marcella for being great friends and second parents to our children; Thad Hyland, Anna Olson, Suzy Johlfs and Merrill Williams and the staff of the Ojai Valley Inn and Spa for their input and support.

About the Authors

Kent Burden has twenty-five years of fitness experience. He is certified as a personal trainer by AFAA and IFPA, as a Pilates instructor, yoga instructor, Spinning instructor, water fitness instructor, systematic touch trainer and massage therapist. As the Mind/Body Program Coordinator at California's famed Ojai Valley Inn and Spa he created the mind and body fitness program that was named by *Spa Finder Magazine* as one of North America's top programs in a field of more than 500 spas. His program is considered to be one of the most innovative and diverse in the industry.

Maria Schell Burden holds a B.A. in American Studies and Spanish from Western Michigan University. In addition to co-authoring *Yin Yang Fitness*, she is the author of *Professor T.S.C. Lowe and his Mountain Railway* and *The Life and Times of Robert G. Fowler* (Borden Publishing). She is certified as a group fitness instructor by AFAA, and as a yoga instructor. Kent and Maria own the fitness consulting firm "My Life Fitness" and are co-creators of the *Essential Triangle*, a mind and body workout that is a union of yoga, Pilates and meditation. The Burdens reside with their children in southern California.

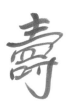

This is the Chinese character for longevity, or long life.
We wish you a healthy and joyful life
and remind you to be present
in this moment and breathe.

CONTENTS

Chapter One: Introduction   1

Chapter Two: Kent's Story   9

Chapter Three: Maria's Story   21

Chapter Four: Nutrition   27

Chapter Five: Meditation and Journaling   39

Chapter Six: Exercise   47

Chapter Seven: Day-by-Day   75

1

INTRODUCTION

Everyone knows that to live a long, productive and satisfying life one must have good health. But what does good health mean to you? Is it a thin body? Is it a muscular body? Is it looking like your favorite movie star? We believe that good health is more than that. Some of today's best-selling books promise to stop the aging process, melt away fat or get you looking great in the buff. But is that enough? We don't think so.

Each of us is a whole package, a series of opposites, checks and balances. Yin and Yang. We are at our best when we are fully in balance. We simply cannot achieve our fullest potential unless we condition the mind and spirit along with the body. If we fail to maintain this balance, the lack of conditioning in one segment of our being will diminish the benefits achieved in another.

A sculpted body controlled by a scattered mind
is worth nothing.

The average American would like a better-looking body, right? Our culture dictates that beautiful bodies and faces are the ultimate goal, and that we should strive for both at any cost. Mind-numbing workouts, dangerous diets, and expensive equipment are the price of being beautiful, the media preaches. And if we don't succeed with exercise, then plastic surgery is the next step. We have been conditioned to be critical of our own bodies and the bodies of others. Competition against oneself and others is a self-defeating exercise that paralyzes the self esteem, overfuels the ego and powers negative self-talk. A cycle of inadequate feelings feeds upon itself and we feel out of control and displeased with ourselves because we aren't a clone of the sixteen year-old models in a fashion magazine.

It is, however, reasonable to wish for better health, and to feel and look your personal best. To exercise for the sole purpose of losing weight is not enough of a reason to sustain the activity regularly for the rest of your life. Your loved ones, you reason, will love you in whatever form your body takes, whether large or slim, fit or unfit. And of course this is true. But you have to desire the tangible benefits of better health to affect real change and sustain it. You must want increased energy levels, improved self esteem, to be with your loved ones as an idependent person able to do the things you want to well into your retirement years without restrictions imposed by poor health.

The greatest griefs are those we cause ourselves.
-Sophacles

Young bodies can take a lot of punishment and still function at an acceptable level. But move the calendar up a few decades. A person who has punished his body throughout youth and middle age, neglected exercise, and made consistently poor food choices will find that his body begins to break down after forty or fifty years. Injuries, chronic conditions and multiple medications lead to restrictions. Life becomes a frightening battle just to stay alive. Who wants to live that way? Wouldn't it be better to start now making healthier choices and avoid playing catch-up later when it may already be too late? If you are in your 40s or 50s or better, it makes sense to regain some of your vitality, flexibility and strength and slow down the aging process.

Yin Yang Fitness will show you how to honor the opposites that make up the whole package that is *you*. You will learn to combine healthy, realistic food choices, cutting-edge fitness without a gym membership, and ancient wisdom into a comprehensive one-hour format. This program can help you achieve sustainable improvements in your health. This is not a fad diet or fad exercise plan for a short-term improvement. This is a life change with effort required. You will have to make time for better health. One hour might sound like an impossible amount of time in your hectic schedule. But if you calculate the time you waste each day waiting in line at a drive-through, talking on the phone or watching television, you will probably find more time than you need to improve your health. And you will have to change some habits.

We never said it would be easy.

The good news is Yin Yang Fitness is time-efficient, reducing the time it takes to be healthy. How much time would it take to drive to the gym, work out, shower and return home? About two hours. If you follow the advice in this book, you can care for your mind, body *and* inner self in about one hour each day. You will never be satisfied with yourself unless you condition your mind and spirit along with your body—until you learn to relax deeply, connect with your source of inner wisdom, and discover *your* personal best, *your* physical, spiritual and mental goals.

A HISTORICAL PERSPECTIVE

Ayurvedic medicine, more than 3,500 years old and one of the most ancient forms of organized medicine, considers good health to be a balance between the physical, mental and spiritual selves. Ayur (life) + veda (knowledge) asserts that soundness of all three elements mind (manas), body (shira) and self (atman) must be present for the individual to experience good health. An ayurvedic practitioner examines the ill patient, asks about the condition of his family life, and if he has prayed that day. According to the principles of Ayurvedic medicine, all of these questions are relevant to your present health. Why? Because our bodies cannot be healthy unless our minds and spirits are equally healthy. If your physician asked about your spiritual health, would you think she was a quack? Ayurvedic practitioners use cooking, diet, yoga, meditation, breathwork, plants and many other elements to guide the individual in achieving this balance. This ancient form of medical practice not only treats illness, but also practices preventive

If your physician asked about your spiritual health, would you think she was a quack?

healthcare and the promotion of healthy habits.

Traditional Chinese Medicine focuses on the balance of yin and yang, of opposites within and without. Like Ayurvedic medicine, Traditional Chinese Medicine emphasizes bringing into balance all components of life to achieve optimum health. Too much focus in one area takes you out of balance, ultimately creating sickness. Yin qualities such as stillness and darkness are opposite Yang qualities such as light and movement. While these qualities are opposites, they are also dependent upon one another. Without its opposite, the other would cease to exist. These qualities must be maintained in harmonious balance. If you were to walk a tightrope while carrying a ten-pound sack of flour in your left hand, you would tip to the left and fall. But if you carried one five-pound sack of flour in each hand you would remain in balance and stay on the tightrope. The same is true of your body.

We live in a contemporary world that seems out of control, technology-driven and overwhelming. Modern medicine focuses a great deal on curing illness with medication and surgery, and very little on prevention. Westerners must consider the huge spikes in incidence of chronic disease, surgical procedures and childhood and adult obesity in determining whether a lack of prevention is really the best form of medicine. We should learn from the wisdom of the ancients and view health from a mind/body perspective, moving people inward so they can be balanced, connected participants in the universe.

A SKEWED VIEW OF HEALTH

Western healthcare is not healthcare at all. It is "sick care." Some insurance companies do not pay for wellness visits, only illness treatment. Physicians are trained to treat illness, but few spend time discussing with patients the benefits of preventive health. Few physicians give nutritional advice, prescribe exercise or inquire about a patient's mental well-being. It seems that the role of western medicine is to prescribe drugs, recommend surgery or refer patients to specialists. This is what they have been trained to do.

The role of this book is not to campaign against the contemporary medical establishment. Medical science performs a vital life-saving service when you are ill. In the case of life-threatening illness or injury, contemporary medical science plays an important role. Regular medical checkups are very important. But good health comes from the things you do every day such as physical exercise, sound food choices and positive mental activity.

Physicians are highly trained and skilled, but they cannot hold your hand every day and remind you to eat properly, sleep, exercise and feed your spirit. A physician cannot force you to see your full potential. You spend less than one hour each year with your physician at a regular checkup. You live a total of 8,760 hours each year. No doctor can impart enough wisdom in a brief annual visit to show you how to avoid unrealistic expectations and goals, destructive thoughts, unhealthy habits and other self-defeating activities in which you might routinely engage.

Every day your body and mind send you important messages and clues you need to take care of yourself and cultivate wellness. You must tune into your mind and body to pick up on the subtle signals—messages of happiness, physical trouble or anxiety. You cannot railroad over these messages and ignore them, because in doing so you miss critical clues to solving problems before they become full-blown conditions that might not be detected by your physician for several years. By then it may be too late for a simple fix. Yin Yang Fitness will show you how to tune in.

You must take responsibility for your own path to wellness. Good health is the result of healthy activities, not some magical place or product. Many people think that if they can just lose 25 pounds, they will be "healthy." Losing weight can be a natural byproduct of a healthy lifestyle, but weight loss by itself is not necessarily good health. People suffering with cancer, anorexia nervosa and bulimia will lose weight, but are they healthy? Of course not.

Once you have tasted good health, energy and confidence, you will find that you instinctively make better choices, have a healthier body image and enjoy feelings of completeness and satisfaction. The real challenge is connecting all the components and maintaining the balance between them. We must combine the wisdom of the ancients and western science to start you down the path to this healthy balance. Through the ancient techniques of visualization, meditation, yoga and controlled breath work, along with modern exercise physiology and nutrition, we will lead you to the discovery of the whole you.

FINDING BALANCE

Talking about balance and actually finding balance in your life are very different things. A client once requested a consultation for her teenage daughter, who we will call Danielle. When Kent first met with Danielle, an athletic girl of sixteen who had worked hard to make the school volleyball team, she expressed frustration with her performance in games, her lack of energy and the appearance of her body, which she termed "fat." She was pale, fatigued, often sick and made frequent technical mistakes during games. Dissatisfied with her performance, she had increased her workouts to seven days a week--a demanding routine that included two hours of cardiovascular exercise, one hour of weight training and two hours of volleyball practice.

Although she was 5'6" and weighed only 120 pounds, she felt fat and had restricted her daily food intake to 1,200 calories. It was no wonder she was sick, lethargic and making technical errors. She was *completely* out of balance, starving her body and mind, and failing to tune into the signals her body was sending. Danielle was headed for crisis.

Kent began to work with her, with a full understanding that volleyball was her first priority. He suggested that her mother schedule an appointment with a therapist to help resolve her unhealthy body image issues. He explained to Danielle that in order to improve her athletic performance, she had to first take care of her mind and body, to bring herself into balance. He recommended two days of rest per week to give her body time to rebuild strength and repair tissue damage. He recommended one hour of cardiopulmonary training five days per week (some of which she was already getting at volleyball practices), one hour of weight training

three days per week, and volleyball practices and games as sched-
uled. A brief yoga/Pilates blend workout rounded out her physical
work. Her very active body, still growing in adolescence, needed *at
least* 2,000 calories per day, perhaps even more.

Kent suggested a consultation with a registered dietician
or nutritionist to help Danielle determine her nutritional needs
and make good choices. In addition to the physical changes to her
routine, she would spend 10 minutes five days per week practic-
ing visualization or meditation. She would visualize herself as strong
and powerful, training her mind to see her body as perfect and
believe it.

Tree Pose

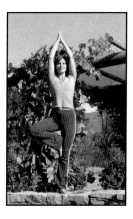

After six months of this routine, Danielle reported feeling
stronger, leaner, more powerful and more in control of her game
and her life. She was learning to pick up the signals her body was
sending, and was experiencing new levels of skill. Because she
had witnessed herself being successful during visualization, she
knew she could be successful. She made contact with--and
strengthened--her inner self. She found balance.

Finding balance in your life is not a goal you will reach,
then bask in its effortless glory. Balance is a never-ending exercise; it is a mental shifting and adjustment, a journey of a thousand miles taken one step at a time.

Try this: Set the book down and stand up. Place your hands
together in prayer position at chest level. Shift your weight to your
left leg. Place the sole of your right foot on the inside of your left
calf or inner thigh. This is a yoga asana (pose) known as Tree. Stand
there for 15 deep breaths, balancing on your left foot. If you want,
raise your hands overhead as shown. Switch legs and repeat the
exercise. You will notice that this balancing exercise is a constant
series of corrections, and that moments of true balance are rare
and fleeting. Enjoy these moments, and feel the joy of getting it,
then make the next correction. Find joy in the moments of success when they come, and they will come more often.

Danielle's story illustrates that each person is unique and
comes from a different background of views on health and fitness.

There is no blanket answer or guideline that will be perfect for everyone. What works for one person may not work for another, and you have to begin to walk your own path to better health. In the next two chapters we will share with you the diversity of our own backgrounds and the paths that led us to create Yin Yang Fitness. Kent's background as an athlete and a fitness natural is a sharp contrast to Maria's past as an unhealthy refugee from fitness. Our goals for fitness and health are quite different, and we each have a different approach with clients because of our varied backgrounds. We are just another example of Yin and Yang—of opposites dependent upon one another for balance.

2

KENT'S STORY

I grew up in the small town of Springfield, Michigan, a white suburb of "cereal city" Battle Creek. For most of my young life I felt like an outsider. Being black, I never felt truly accepted by my predominantly white schoolmates; being very light-skinned, I was never truly accepted in the black community. As an only child, I had no siblings to relate to. The only place I understood my role was on the athletic field. From the time I was in elementary school I played daily football, basketball, baseball and any other games you can imagine. Most times I played with kids several years older than I was: each Sunday, I played football with a group of varsity and junior varsity players from the high school. Even though I was the youngest, I was always among the first selected when teams were chosen—a true boost to any kid's ego.

I went from sandlot hero to playing organized sports in junior high school, where I broke records: most touchdowns in a football season, most points scored in a basketball game and longest long jump in track. My little league coaches chose me for the all-star game each year. I was a powerhouse in sports.

Yet socially, I felt inferior—not part of any group, I had few close friends. I tried hard to fit in and be liked. I even lied about my race and made up elaborate stories about my racial composition, but I was just hanging on the social fringe.

By the time I reached high school, I was very aware that

my social standing directly correlated to achievement in athletics. So I trained hard and pushed myself to be better. I learned everything I could about nutrition, weight training and cardiovascular stamina and read books by great champions. I listened to coaches and broadcasters trying to extract grains of wisdom to gain an edge over my rival athletes.

But at an age when a kid just wants to be like everyone else, I wasn't. There were only seven blacks at Springfield high school and I didn't even look like them, nor did I look like the whites. I looked different. And I was interested in music, art and theater, none of which scored major points in my social circle. So I ignored what I loved and let my entire sense of self-worth revolve around my athletic performance. I believed that people would like me and respect me if I were a better athlete. But no matter what I achieved, the fathers who cheered me on each Friday night at the football games forbade their daughters to go out with me on Saturday night.

I lettered in four sports each year of high school, then went on to play football for Saginaw Valley State University. It was both

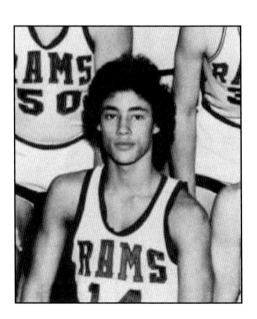

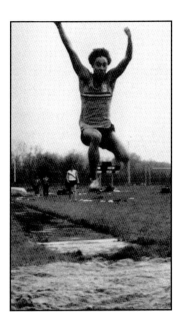

heaven and hell. Playing college football had always been my dream. It enforced my sense of self-worth, since I knew people back home were following my athletic career. But college football put intense importance on winning: losing seasons could cost staff member's jobs and the athletes felt the pressure. As a wide receiver, spectacular catches were expected of me- so I sacrificed my body to the defensive backs during each practice, hoping for a place in the starting lineup.

At the end of my freshman year the coach told me that I would have to gain at least twenty pounds of muscle if I hoped to contend for a starting position the following fall. During that off-season I chugged weight gain shakes, pumped heavy iron three or four times per week, researched strength training and pored over *Pumping Iron,* but nothing worked. Desperate, I started taking anabolic steroids, which is incredibly stupid. (I mention it here to show how entirely my self-esteem was attached to my athletic performance.) After five months of hard work and stupidity, I went back to college the next fall and won that coveted playing time. I had a great second season, played explosively and made a name for myself on the playing field, which felt level for the first time in my life. By the end of my sophomore year, my body had matured naturally as well, so I no longer needed the steroids to compete with the big boys. After a long off-season of hard training, I returned to the field with high hopes for a great year...and more than a little bit of arrogance.

During the first game, I was sprinting across the field for a reception when another player slammed his helmeted head like a battering ram into the center of my lower back. After the hit I got up feeling stiff, but played the rest of the game. On the bus trip home my back hurt, but that wasn't unusual. Later in my dorm room, my back muscles began to spasm. In an attempt to relax the muscles, I got down on the floor to stretch. I felt something tear and heard a loud crack, *and everything from my chest down went dead.*

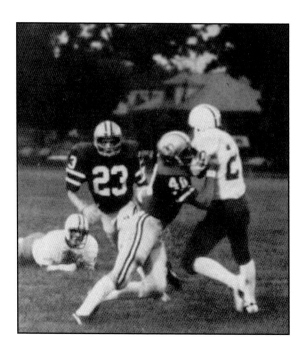

I lay there in the dark on the floor. No feeling, no movement. Nothing. I convinced myself that I wasn't scared: a few weeks earlier, a "stinger," or pinched nerve in my neck had left one arm numb and useless for several hours. I told myself that this was the same thing.

I woke up my roommate, who called the trainers. Bleary-eyed, they arrived at my room and checked my legs for reflexes-but found none. They exchanged nervous glances as one of them called an ambulance.

After hours of X-rays and a battery of other tests, a doctor came to my bedside.

"I have some bad news," he began.

With the arrogance of youth, I finished his sentence inside my head: *You're out for the season, son.* I prepared myself, knowing I should take it like a man. How would I deal with being on the sidelines for an entire season? What would my coach say?

The doctor's next words made those questions seem trivial.

"You've crushed two disks and cracked the vertebrae in between. Pieces of the disks have shifted into the spinal cord, putting pressure on it. There's a great deal of swelling. You may walk again in an hour. You may never walk again. We honestly don't know."

The rest of the doctor's speech fell on deaf ears. I didn't know what to say, or what to do. Too numb to make a decision, I cried myself to sleep that night, alone in a hospital room hundreds of miles from home.

The next few days were a waiting game to see if the swelling would go down so the doctors could determine the extent of the damage to my spinal column. I had never been so devastated; just one week earlier I had made a spectacular catch in front of thousands of screaming fans. Now I couldn't even move my legs.

My hospital roommate was a young quadriplegic man, the victim of a motorcycle accident five years before. He was in the hospital because his caregiver had placed him in too-hot bath water; neither of them had realized until his skin turned bright red. I imagined myself in his place.

One night as we lay talking in the glow from the television screen, he told me not to give up hope. "With hard work, you can make progress." With extreme effort he lifted his hand two inches off the bed, then almost imperceptibly wiggled his fingers. He smiled and dropped his hand back down with a tired sigh.

"I've worked three years to do that," he said proudly. Then, exhausted, he fell asleep.

Christ, I thought to myself, *the poor guy can't even lift his hand to wipe his own brow.* Later, I called my best buddy at the college and asked him to sneak me a pint of Southern Comfort. I drank myself to sleep that night.

You can run, but you cannot hide; This is widely known.
-James Taylor

I spent the next nine months in a wheelchair, waiting to see if I would ever walk again. Each morning I woke up hoping for a tingle in my toes. My entire self-worth had revolved around what I could do with my body; people used to look up to me. Now they looked down on me—literally. This was the darkest period of my life. Deeply depressed, I began to abuse prescription drugs and alcohol. I dropped out of school and brooded.

But even this dark and difficult time had a silver lining: I re-evaluated my priorities and asked myself what I really wanted to do with my life. While I had never really thought I would play professional football, I'd never given any thought to what I would do when my college football career came to an end.

Well, it had come to an end all right.

The first thing I admitted to myself was that I had made a mistake by majoring in engineering. It had been the college "major *du jour"* and I had joined the crowd with total disregard for the fact that my mathematics aptitude was in the basement. Accepting that I would never excel at such a technical field, I began to ask myself some tough questions during those long, sleepless nights. "If someone gave you a job making $100,000 a year to do something that bored you for ten hours a day, five days per week, would that make you happy?"

I knew that it wouldn't. But I was desperate for happiness.

Not just pleasure, but true, fulfilling, thrilled-down-to-your-toes, happiness! Unfortunately I didn't know where to look for it.

The Mind-Body Connection

It was during this period that I began to remember the advice of my high school drama teacher, Jeanne Grandstaff: "Find something you love to do. If you do something you love, the money will follow." I took her words to heart, as well as other things she had talked about: meditation, visualization, the connection between the body and the mind. I learned about meditation, mantras, creative visualization, breathing techniques and concentration meditations. I read stories about Tibetan monks who could raise their body temperatures at will. I read stories about great yogis who could slow their heart rates and breathing to a level so low that doctors declared them dead. But most importantly, I learned of people finding great inner peace and insight.

At first I had to battle my own skepticism, but I figured I had nothing to lose. Learning to meditate was incredibly difficult for me; I was deemed "hyperactive" as a child, and my wife Maria and I suspect, although I have never been diagnosed, that I suffer from Attention Deficit Disorder. But I persisted, and eventually my chattering brain began to quiet itself. I began to experiment with visualization and other positive imaging techniques. I saw myself setting the brakes on my wheelchair and standing up. I watched myself walk effortlessly down a beach. These mental "vacations" were therapeutic, and I found myself taking more and more of them. My depression began to lift as I saw myself doing all kinds of everyday things. I stopped thinking privately "*If* I ever walk again...," and began saying aloud, "*When* I can walk again..." The power of these positive images and affirmations was remarkable.

For the next nine months I meditated, did physical therapy, and waited to see if the swelling in my spine would go down. During that time, I summoned the courage to return to college in my wheelchair. My plan to make that triumphant return on two strong legs would just have to wait until my body cooperated. I began taking a diverse selection of classes: music history, economics, physical education, philosophy, theater and political science, searching for what interested me.

During my first semester back at school, the doctors finally decided the swelling in my spine would never go down without intervention. If I wanted a chance to walk again, I would need major surgery. And there was the possibility that it wouldn't work.

During spring break, while my fellow students were participating in beer chugging contests with scantily clad coeds in Fort Lauderdale, I underwent hours of surgery. They removed the two damaged disks and fragments of debris, then fused the vertebrae.

For two days nothing happened.

On the third morning, I awoke to searing pain—shooting down both of my legs. It hurt like hell, but the tears rolling down my cheeks were from joy, not pain. Unable to speak, I watched as my toes moved up and down at my bidding. I had been given a second chance to walk, and I could hardly wait to start.

But the muscles in my midsection and legs had atrophied severely during their nine-month hiatus. My body weight had dropped from a hearty 185 pounds to a scrawny 140 and my legs looked like withered sticks.

Even so, I was mentally ready for the long journey back to physical fitness. My doctors started me out in the pool, walking from one end to the other using a walker with the physical therapist supporting me. Progress was slow at first: it took me a long time just to lift one foot, then set it down again. But after while, it took me less and less time to walk across that pool, until finally my therapist confided that I had made the fastest progress of anyone he'd seen. He asked: "Why do you always close your eyes when you start to walk?"

"Because I'm not walking," I told him. "I'm running. I'm big and strong and running so fast that clumps of dirt and grass are flying behind me. The earth simply can't stand up to the powerful force I'm creating."

I even visualized myself playing football again. I could hear and see the standing ovation from the crowd, see myself and my teammates line up for the first play: the center to the quarterback, who fakes a handoff to the halfback. Then the quarterback takes a two-step drop and lofts the ball into the air. I run past the defensive back like he's standing still; the ball floats gracefully, then I reach up and feel it strike my hands. I pull it in and run effortlessly into the end zone.

Then I simply drop the ball and wall back to the locker room without looking back. I never wanted to play again; but the point of my visualization was to prove to myself that I COULD if I wanted to.

Visualization got me through some tough times. When I regained the feeling in my legs and torso, I was in a lot of pain because the muscles were atrophied and tight. Everything had to be strengthened and stretched. The strengthening was hard, but the stretching was pure agony!

The visualizations also helped me through a regimen of core stabilizer exercises that I came, years later, to know as Pilates. The Pilates strengthened the muscles in my midsection and back, helping me to hold myself erect, and the breathing exercises associated with it helped me focus on what I was doing.

Still, at the beginning everything was a struggle, as my mind had to teach my legs how to make even the most basic movements. Physical therapy was a painful reminder of how far I still had to go. Attending classes with a walker and seeing the looks of pity from former teammates and fellow students was enough to make me want to hide in my dorm room. But overcoming each obstacle gave me a sense of forward motion. One full year of intense physical therapy brought progress from wheelchair to walker to a cane, and finally walking unaided.

I would never be the athlete I had once been, but I was walking. And even more than that, I had discovered something about myself and something about life. My identity as a sports hero was gone forever, but I had reached inside myself and found that sports was not my only outlet for self-expression. I was more than just a body on an athletic field. Those early, life-changing events shaped my thoughts and visions, and led to the path I would travel.

Shortly after college, I married my best friend and soul mate, Maria Schell. More than twenty years have passed since my injury, and we live in California with our son and daughter. Health and fitness have become my life's work. I am the mind-body program coordinator at the Ojai Valley Inn and Spa. There I teach classes in yoga, Pilates, the Essential Triangle, spinning, water aerobics, and also serve as a personal trainer.

For many years I convinced myself that what I had been through hadn't been all that bad. I didn't want to think about it too much; I would just work hard and share my knowledge of fitness with others. Then one day, a student challenged me.

The soothing spiritual setting of the Ojai Valley has an uncanny way of bringing people a sense of clarity that helps them articulate their needs and issues. On this particular day, the fall air was crisp and the ground was dry, covered with oak leaves forming a blanket on the soft grass outside the studio. I decided to hold my Essential Triangle class out in the sunlight and clean air. The participants seemed normal enough: a mix of women, with one who had more difficulty than the others achieving certain poses. After class, she waited (defiantly, I thought), then approached me, a distinctive limp marring her walk.

"During class," she said, "I was thinking that it must be easy for you to tell someone to push herself and work hard—a pretty boy like you probably hasn't seen a tough day in his life. Then, as you were demonstrating the downward-facing dog pose, I caught a glimpse of that six-inch scar on your spine. How is it," she asked "that you are even standing here talking to me? It must be a pretty amazing story—you should have told the class."

That one student convinced me not to keep my story to myself, but to share it with anyone who needed to hear it. For some people, my story helps to bring minor problems into perspective. For others with severe physical challenges, my story illustrates that if I can walk and have a highly physical career, then maybe they can achieve their goals, too.

And as much as it helps others, it helps me, too. As a forty-one year old man whose back has been described by most physicians as a "train wreck," I can honestly say that the daily exercise, meditation and healthy diet at the heart of my work is what keeps me on my feet. The incredible flexibility in my joints can only be explained as a benefit of my daily regimen.

That I have been blessed with the opportunity to be physical for a living is remarkable. That strangers benefit from that work is exciting. That I also benefit is exhilarating, and no small miracle.

3

MARIA'S STORY

I was born in Royal Oak, Michigan, the youngest of five children. When I was nearly three, my parents learned that I had asthma. In the mid-1960s there was no preventive asthma medication. My attacks were frequent and severe, and by the age of five my lungs were already damaged. The doctors warned my parents that I would probably not live a long, normal life.

Throughout my childhood asthma controlled my family. We had to give away our family cat when the doctors decided that cat dander might be a problem. It didn't help. Instead of sharing a room with my older sisters, I had to sleep in my own room with sparse furnishings where dust could be minimized and my already-busy mother could sterilize things daily. I was afraid of the dark and hated being alone at night, but because the doctors insisted, we followed orders. It didn't help.

During family vacations I ended up sick with asthma. Out of necessity my mother became an amateur pharmacist, researching the latest developments and medications. The drugs of the day made me jittery, nauseous, pale and weak. None of them helped my condition. During the most severe attacks, doctors administered painful cortisone injections, trying unsuccessfully to reduce the inflammation in my lungs. Common cold viruses kept me out of school for weeks, and my immune system was so weak that I caught every bug that came along. I even had scarlet fever twice (*normal* people only got it once). I was anything but normal.

Physical education classes at school were the ultimate proof of my physical limitations. Whistle-blowing, competition-oriented teachers pointed out the inadequacies in my performance, and I became afraid to participate at all.

"I can't," became my personal mantra.

I manipulated the system so I would be safe from criticism, finding ways to participate only in things that I knew would not put me at risk. I came to believe in my limitations more than my abilities.

Fifteen years of weekly allergy shots garnered no measurable results. I was a teenage refugee of the medical establishment and had come to the conclusion that nothing I did made any difference. Without the strength and support of my parents and siblings, and their resolve to make me well, I might have given into the temptation to escape with drugs and alcohol. My mother, determined that my life be as normal as possible, encouraged me to

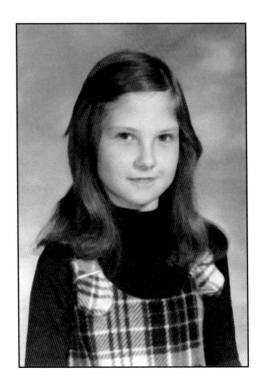

try new things regardless of the risks. She led my Girl Scout troop for more than ten years and took us camping and traveling to far-off places. She was always nearby, and we dealt with the asthma attacks when they came. If she hadn't put so much effort into my life, I would not have been able to try anything new.

At seventeen, I left home to attend college 150 miles away on an academic scholarship. I resolved that asthma would neither limit my success nor control my life. I felt good most of the time, and enjoyed life as a *normal* person without labels, restrictions and self-doubt. I felt strong and smart and ready to attack life with gusto.

I met Kent on a blind date arranged by a mutual friend. His great sense of humor and easygoing nature were therapeutic. He proved to me time and again that I could do anything I set my mind to. We became inseparable. His life as an only child became a life full of brothers, brothers-in-law, sisters and sisters-in-law. He liked being part of a large family where one is never alone. I enjoyed the peace and quiet of being with just him, a soothing balance. We moved in together one year later and have been together ever since. He didn't buy my excuses for not being physically active. He taught me to play tennis, raquetball and lift weights. He became my defacto personal trainer. How could I argue with a recovered paraplegic who lifted weights, played softball, intramural football and golf!

We married after college and Kent's career took us to Los Angeles, California. We had two children in three years and were struggling to make ends meet. Both kids were born with asthma. My own asthma faded into the background in the warm, dry California climate. I was occasionally reminded of it when I caught a cold or other virus, but ignored my doctor's suggestions that I try the new preventive inhalers. I was too busy taking care of everyone else.

Stress, too little sleep, and a lot of responsibility began to take its toll. We were living in the San Gabriel Valley, an area known for high temperatures and heavy smog during the summer. One

*Whether you think
you can
or you can't,
you are right.
-Henry Ford*

June we all got chicken pox. Our four year old son was admitted to the hospital with respiratory complications.

I had a mild case—only a few tiny marks—and was declared uncontagious, so I stayed at the hospital days and nights with our son. After three days I went home for a rest and woke up a few hours later in severe respiratory distress. My asthma was completely out of control. I was rushed to the hospital and admitted. A day later Kent brought our little boy to my room—he had just been released from the pediatric ward of the same hospital.

As my son hugged and kissed me my heart tumbled. He and his baby sister needed me, but I was fading away. I no longer had the strength to force oxygen into my lungs, and I knew that if it were up to me to continue breathing on my own, I would die. With no measurable lung capacity, I struggled to say what was on my mind as Kent moved the oxygen mask aside: "I love you," and "Is my life insurance paid up?" He ran for the nurse, and within an hour I was intubated and hooked to a respirator with machines keeping me alive.

Family members flew in from across the country, and for days they waited, praying that chicken pox had not actually invaded my lungs—a fatal complication that causes them to fill with fluid.

Several days later I became aware of voices in my room. People were talking about me and I struggled to open my Morphine-sleepy eyes. The first things I saw were the faces of my family looking down at me. "I must have died," my muddled mind suggested, thinking they were looking into my casket. Then someone said "She's waking up." The tube in my throat was torture. I made a writing gesture, and Kent handed me pen and paper.

"The babies?" I scribbled. Kent assured me that they were fine. "How are you?" he asked.

"O.K." I scrawled in the biggest letters I could manage. I knew that I would be okay. I would come home to them and take better care of myself so that I would always be there for them. I could not see my children for several days; the superhighway of tubes coming in and out of my body would have been too frightening.

After being released from the hospital, I just wanted things to be normal again. But our life would never be the same. My voice was damaged from the respirator tube forced between my vocal cords, and nighttime lullabies came out raspy. The kids were frightened that I would go away again and never come back. As I healed, Kent and I resolved to make some changes that would improve our lives and health. We soon left behind the smog and heat of the San Gabriel Valley, the stresses of my Los Angeles commute and high-pressure job, and put our family's health first. We moved to the coast, far north of the city where the air is clean and the pace is slower.

The Yoga Connection

For years Kent had suggested that I try yoga. He explained that yoga focuses on effective breathing—sure to benefit my condition. I was ready to go for it now. I explored yogic breathing and was surprised to learn that I had been breathing ineffectively all my life. As an asthmatic child struggling to breathe, I hunched my back and hyper-expanded my chest with each breath. Those ineffective breathing patterns had stayed with me into adulthood. Yogic breathing taught me to use my diaphragm to fully open and expand my lungs. It exercised and strengthened my lungs and greatly improved their function.

Kent taught me a basic sun salutation series with a variety of asanas to improve posture and flexibility and I began to practice almost every day. My love of yoga was born of this simple beginning—and changed my perception of my own abilities. "I can't" became "I can and I will."

Today I am a mind and body fitness professional with certifications in group fitness and yoga. I teach yoga and the Essential Triangle, I write fiction and nonfiction, and take care of my family and myself. Our children have a new respect for me because I honor them by caring for my body and mind.

The physical and emotional scars remain, but they are evidence of the path I took to the beautiful here and now. The scars remind me to simply be here in this moment, and breathe.

4

NUTRITION

Webster's dictionary defines nutrition, in part as "the series of processes by which an organism takes in and assimilates food for promoting growth and replacing worn or injured tissues. " This definition sheds light on the important role nutrition—not diet—plays in your healthy body. We are bombarded by messages about "dieting" to lose weight. Our focus in this book is not simply about weight loss. Scientific research clearly shows that being overweight is detrimental to good health and increases our risk of developing coronary heart disease, some types of cancer, diabetes, hypertension, joint problems, and many other health problems. The Centers for Disease Control and Prevention estimate that more than half of the American population is overweight. This number increases each year. More than twenty-two percent of Americans are obese. This number has risen significantly in the past twenty years. To ignore the issue of obesity would be irresponsible. To be obese *and* inactive is the most dangerous combination of all. To bring about real change, we must take a hard look at what we eat, and how much we eat.

The old axiom "you are what you eat" is trite but true. Most Americans are used to feeling overly full and lethargic because they consume diets high in saturated fat and excess calories, inadequate amounts of fresh produce and whole grains. Many people have no idea that they could feel better if they made some simple changes in food selection. The other problem with American eating habits is portion size. Portions are, well—huge. Americans in particular believe that more is somehow better. So we eat more; we clean our plates no matter how high the pile of food! Many people are used to feeling full instead of satisfied. Full means overfed. As the stomach stretches to accommodate this over-feeding, the body demands more food to achieve that feeling of fullness. Large portions translate to large calorie counts; large calorie counts translate to large bodies. See "Portion Size" later in this chapter.

We do not advocate quick fixes or crash diets. We advocate good healthy foods in portions large enough to fuel the body with enough calories to sustain the energy that will be used over the course of a day. If you take the time to improve your nutrition, it will show in your energy level and appearance. It will help create a positive change in your self-image. Better nutrition creates harmony within your body.

There are hundreds of diet and nutrition books on the market today. Many books promise to help you lose weight, keep cancer at bay or boost energy levels. Like Yin Yang Fitness, most of them are twelve-week plans. These books promise miraculous results in the first few weeks—if you buy their expensive proprietary brand foods in the form of shakes, nutrition bars or both. Others promise these results, but require that you dedicate several hours per day to exercise, complicated menus, hard-to-find foods and calorie counting that a tax analyst couldn't understand. Yes, better health does require a commitment and some time, but it is unrealistic to spend several hours per day working out, shopping and cooking and still live your real life. You need tools to balance real life and good health. We will give you those tools and show you that it is all about balance.

Nutrition is a critical component of Yin Yang Fitness. You can jog five miles each day, play tennis on the weekends and swim laps at the pool every day, but if you are eating processed meal replacement bars for two of your three meals each day, you are not in good balance or good health. The only way to eat properly is to plan carefully and use whole foods whenever possible.

It is our belief that nutrition is simple. There are no magic bullets. There is no food bar or supplement or energy drink that will deliver good health without effort. If you want to feel and look better, you need to start now changing how you eat. Make at least one healthy change per day, say eating half of the skin of your baked potato instead of just scooping out the center—that can add as much as 1.5 grams of fiber to a serving depending on the size of the potato. Learn to look for opportunities for improved nutrients at every meal or snack.

WHOLE FOODS

What is whole food? Whole food is food that has not been unnecessarily processed. Artificial colors and flavors, or ingredients and words on a label that you cannot pronounce are all signs that a food is not whole. Bleached white flour (whole wheat flour with the nutrients and fiber strained and bleached out of it) is not a whole food. Go back a few steps in the evolution of white bread and buy the whole-wheat flour, or the loaf of bread that lists whole-wheat flour as its first ingredient. Eat fresh fruits and vegetables whenever possible. The next best choice would be frozen, then canned as the last resort. Legumes, beans of all colors, and brown rice (white rice is bleached and contains almost no fiber) are only a few of the many high-fiber choices out there. Whole foods are often lower in calories than processed foods, which means that you can eat more of them, get more nutrients, and feel fuller. Whole foods pack more nutritional value for your calories than processed foods and will give you a greater sustained energy source too.

The only way to make sense out of change is to plunge into it, move with it, and join the dance.
-Alan Watts

FRESH FRUITS AND VEGETABLES

The single most important change you can make that will have a positive comprehensive effect is eating seven to ten servings of fresh fruits and vegetables per day. According to the Produce for Better Health Foundation, which has created and popularized the "5 a day for better health" slogan, people should eat at least five servings per day. We don't think that is enough. We think that seven to ten servings per day are better. Fresh fruits and vegetables are a great source of fiber, vitamins, minerals and trace elements, which can protect your heart and other organs from damage and keep your body functioning at its best.

So, how much is a serving size of fruits or vegetables? Here are some examples from the 5-a-day for Better Health Foundation:

One medium-size fruit

$^3/_4$ cup (6 oz.) of 100 percent fruit or vegetable juice

$^1/_2$ cup canned vegetables or fruit

1 cup of raw leafy vegetables

$^1/_2$ cup cooked dry peas or beans

$^1/_4$ cup dried fruit

So start now eating a large variety of fruits and vegetables, whole grains, high-fiber low fat foods from as close to the source (whole foods—not processed) as you can possibly get.

BUYING ADVICE: PLANNING = SUCCESS

Eating well is about preparing well. Create a weekly menu, (manyhealthy recipes are available on our website, www.mylifefitness.com) then choose healthy snack options and buy accordingly. This strategy makes it easier to eat a balanced diet without having to spend an eternity putting it together each day. This will also make it easier to be successful at being healthy. The most common pitfall is having an excuse to fall out of good eating habits. If you've run out of healthy foods and the box of Twinkies for your kid's lunch is the first thing you see when you open the cupboard, you'll be more tempted to eat one, right?

Most people work outside the home and many of us are raising families too. Yes, you are busy, but you probably go to the grocery store at least a few times each week. Take an extra five minutes and pick up a few things from the produce aisle to replenish your produce supplies.

If you eat meat, buy lean cuts of meat in small amounts. Divide the meat into three-ounce servings and freeze them individually. In prehistoric times, animals were lean because they ran all the time. Today's meat is cultivated to be flavorful, so it is higher in fat. Since we are significantly less active than our caveman ancestors, this is a bad combination. We don't advocate a vegetarian diet unless this suits you. It does not suit us. We enjoy lean meat and fish in small portions along with fresh vegetables and fruits.

Whole foods can be readily found in the *average* grocery store where most of us shop. Some whole foods like whole wheat pasta and high-fiber breads can cost more than their less nutritious mainstream shelfmates, but they are worth it. Improving your nutrition is a lifestyle change worth making. People do not undertake lifestyle changes for frivolous reasons. You wouldn't sell all your belongings and move to a monastery because of a disappointing annual job review. Nor would you sell your home and move to a distant corner of the world just because you didn't like the color of the living room walls. You make lifestyle changes for compelling reasons—things that are truly important; improving your health is a vitally important lifestyle change that permeates all aspects of your life.

VARIETY

Humans are creatures of habit. But try not to buy the same fruits and vegetables week after week. If you don't vary your diet, you will miss out on vitamins and minerals in new foods. Try to have lots of different produce around the house. Keep long-lasting staples on hand too, like carrots and sweet potatoes, so that when your other varieties are depleted and you can't get to the store you will still have a healthy option. Remember, don't give yourself an excuse to eat the bad stuff. With every meal or snack over the course of the day, eat a different fruit or vegetable. Take a stroll down your fresh produce aisle and pick up something you haven't tried before. There are some great vegetable cookbooks on the market. Give something new a try. While waiting in line at

the checkout, flip through one of the many health and fitness magazines on display—recipes and nutrition tips abound. Buy one per
week. You'll find that just reading it will inspire you to try new
things and make better choices.

COLOR

Make an effort to bring color to your meals. The more color
you bring to you plate, the healthier the meal. Yellow, green, red,
orange purple and blue bring different nutrients to your body. And
of course, they look beautiful on the plate. A beautiful plate is a
healthy plate.

HIGH-FIBER FOODS

High-fiber foods help us in a number of ways. High-fiber
foods will help you feel full more quickly so you are less likely to
eat more calories than your body needs. Fiber also cleanses your
digestive tract, helping your digestive system to work more efficiently. Since fiber is more difficult to digest than other foods, you
burn more calories by simply digesting it.

A low-fiber diet contributes to constipation, bowel irregu-
larity and increased risk of bowel diseases like colon cancer. The
recommended daily intake of dietary fiber is 25 to 35 grams. According to a study by the University of Iowa, the average American
adult consumes only 10 to12 grams of fiber per day. This is a critical deficit that can have serious health implications. A high-fiber
diet not only promotes bowel regularity, it can also reduce the risk
of breast, colon, and other cancers by as much as 40%. Studies
also show that in many people fiber helps reduce cholesterol and
stabilize blood glucose levels.

So, where is fiber? Fiber is found in whole grain breads,
cereals, fresh fruits, vegetables and legumes. Super fiber sources
that are easy to find include black beans and blueberries.

Americans have become accustomed to diets high in simple
carbohydrates. Over the past century food has become "white."
In order to make whole grains look white and refined, they must be
excessively processed, which unfortunately removes the best nutrients. Simple carbohydrates are found in white bread, bagels,

sweetened breakfast cereals, mashed potatoes, white rice, boxed macaroni and cheese, pasta, packaged snack cakes, cookies and crackers—sound familiar? Your pantry may be full of them. These simple carbohydrates convert quickly into simple sugars, cause your insulin level to spike, and force your body to store these sugars as fat. These foods throw your body chemistry *out of balance*. The complex carbohydrates in high-fiber foods break down slowly and efficiently, releasing steady energy and nutrients over a long period. Complex carbohydrates make you feel satisfied longer.

What is a simple carbohydrate as opposed to a complex carbohydrate? Complex carbohydrates are grains or starches that have not been unnecessarily processed or refined and include whole wheat flour, oats in many forms, brown rice, wild rice, couscous, bulgur, beans, whole potatoes (including the skin) and many others.

Our advice: don't buy anything without first checking the nutrition label. Learn to zero in on the "dietary fiber" listing on the nutrition label in breads, pastas and cereals. If a product has less than 2 grams of fiber per serving, pass on it. Try for 3 or more grams of fiber per serving—it will make a difference in how you feel. Many brands of whole wheat bread found in chain grocery stores are very high in fiber. You just have to choose the right ones. Healthy foods might cost more money than some overly processed foods. Wonder bread (with 0 grams of fiber per serving) costs less than a loaf of Ezekiel bread that has three to five grams of fiber for every slice. Remember that whole foods are the fuel of your healthy new body. Just as you wouldn't put low-quality fuel in a racecar and expect peak performance, you should not put low-quality fuel in your body and expect to feel good.

PORTION SIZE

How much you eat is just as important as what you eat. In America, we have a distorted view of proper portions. Super Size has become a way of life—large is now the standard at many fast food restaurants. Unfortunately, this is reflected in the size of our bodies. Pay attention to the portion size on nutrition labels. Measure it out at first until you get used to what a reasonable portion looks like.

Restaurants are the most difficult places to keep a handle on portion size. We feel that we are getting a good value if we are presented with enormous portions of food and we feel obligated to finish everything. For generations parents told children to finish everything on their plate because there were starving children in China. We must realize that obesity can be just as deadly as malnutrition. Get used to noticing when you are *satisfied*, not full. Note the moment when you no longer feel hungry. That is the satisfaction point. When you feel *full*, you have actually overeaten, and by the time your brain receives the signal from your stomach that it is full, it is overly full. When you first feel satisfied, stop eating and get used to leaving that remaining food on your plate.

The chief object of education is not to learn things but to unlearn things.
-G.K. Chesterton

If you feel obligated to finish everything on your plate in a restaurant, try this: when you order your meal, ask that half of your meal be put in a carryout container before being brought to the table. Then, you won't be staring at the other half of the sandwich and thinking that you don't want it to go to waste. This is especially important for people who travel on business and eat almost every meal in a restaurant.

Beverages are also super-size. A serving of soda is about twelve ounces. Just because fast-food restaurants are serving up 42-ounce sodas in a cup so large you could bathe a small child in it doesn't mean you have to drink the whole thing and go back for refills. Soda is loaded with refined sugar (a simple carbohydrate just waiting to turn into fat).

WHEN TO EAT

We recommend that you eat several small meals over the course of the day. This practice helps your body stay fueled all day long. A steady high-quality fuel supply means no insulin spikes and no moments of feeling ravenous, which is when bingeing is most likely to occur. Balanced nutrition, balanced portions, balanced timing. We suggest that you eat four to six small meals per day, and try to eat every two to three hours during the day. Three of these "meals" are really just healthy snacks. Snacking after dinner is not a good idea unless you snack on something healthy like fruit or vegetables. If you are trying to lose weight, we suggest that you stop eating three hours before bedtime.

CALORIES

There was a time when popular thinking was forget about calories and count only fat grams. Those days are gone. Calories do count. If you eat more calories than your body can burn, your body will convert those calories to fat stores and you *will* gain weight.

Generally, women should eat 1800-2200 calories per day, and men should eat 2,000-2500 calories per day. These are approximate figures. If you are a woman who is five feet tall and less than one hundred pounds, 1,800 calories may be too high for you. On the other hand, a man who is more than six feet tall with 250 pounds of muscle probably needs more than 2,500 calories per day. If in doubt, consult a dietician. How do you know what your ideal caloric intake should be?

Keep it in balance. You and your body must learn to be satisfied consuming the correct number of calories. A 1,200-calorie diet cannot sustain your body and support good health for long. You might be able to starve yourself for a week or two, but you will either become ill, or you will swing radically to the other extreme and binge because you are starving. You will gain back all of the weight you lost, plus a few pounds. Starving yourself on 1,200 calories a day does not teach you to eat real food in real portions. Crash diets are not balanced. Remember, Yin Yang Fitness is all about balance. You can do this.

Each person's metabolism is different, so these numbers are approximate. An average American who is overweight and does not currently monitor their calorie intake is almost *certainly* taking in too many calories. Another way to determine your optimal calorie intake is by watching and listening to your own body. If you are gaining fat, you are probably taking in too many calories. At any weight if you begin to feel tired, lethargic and constantly hungry, you may not be getting enough calories, or your calories may be coming from the wrong balance of sources. These nutritional improvements are changes you will make for the rest of your life; this is not a diet for a limited time, so you have to learn to create a balance that you can live with. Take the time to listen to your body. It is worth doing. Experiment with the amount of food your body needs to feel good, and what kind of food makes you feel energized and well.

How important is food to your good health? It is very important. In both Chinese and Ayurvedic medicine doctors treat illness with food. These forms of medicine have been practiced for thousands of years with remarkable success. Ancient cultures can teach us that what we eat makes a huge impact on the quality and length of our lives. A balanced diet keeps the body in balance, helps the spirit remain strong and keeps the mind agile and supple. The best way to be healthy is to stop sickness, disease and other destructive forces that prey upon the human body before they can start. Eating a healthy, balanced diet can do that.

Even stronger "medicine" would be to add exercise and visualization/meditation to this potent prescription for good health. How many times have you either skipped breakfast or eaten a huge fatty breakfast and felt lousy for the rest of the day? Because you felt "out of sorts" you were cranky and lethargic. Maybe you decided *not* to do something that you normally enjoy, which left you in an even deeper funk. These negative physical and emotional feelings carry throughout your day and can build upon one another until a pattern of inactivity develops. Does your diet affect your balance and emotional well-being? It absolutely does.

WATER

Just as important as making healthy food choices is keeping your body hydrated. Drinking pure, clean water often throughout each day is an important component of good health. Both eastern medicine and western science agree that without adequate hydration our body cannot function properly. How much water is enough? That depends upon the individual but a good rule is to drink sixty-four ounces (that is eight eight-ounce glasses) per day. Many of us mistake hunger for thirst, so drinking this quantity of water each day can help you avoid overeating. Adequate water intake also flushes toxins from the body. Sodas and juice drinks are high-calorie items, so consume them sparingly.

PROTEIN

High-quality complete protein is another key component to a balanced, healthy diet. This is especially important since Yin Yang Fitness includes strength training and your body needs protein to build muscle tissue and maintain energy levels. The best protein source is fish, which is low in fat and high in protein. The fat found in fish is actually what scientists today call "good fat" containing omega three fatty acids. The next best source is lean poultry or red meat. Depending on your size and weight you should keep your total intake of fish, poultry or lean meat between three to six ounces two to four times per week. If you do include fish or meat in your diet every day, we recommend no more than three to six ounces two to three times per week. Keep your intake of saturated fats low and hydrogenated fats to a bare minimum. When eating fat, try for the good fats like olive oil, canola oil and the omega three fatty acids found in fish. By experimenting with your diet, you will find the amounts that will make you feel your best.

If you are a vegetarian, be sure to eat plenty of beans and rice (the only combination that rivals the protein found in meat) and soy-based products on a regular basis. These foods will deliver the amino acids and trace elements your body needs to stay healthy.

FOOD IS FUEL

When preparing for weekend backpacking trips as kids, our scoutmaster used to tell us "don't carry more than you can eat." By the same token, do not eat more than you can burn. Eat because you are hungry, not because you are sad, angry, bored or depressed. Food is fuel; it is not a crutch.

Realistically, you cannot eat perfectly every day. But if you could do it 85% of the time, wouldn't that be better than what you're doing now?

Because it is difficult to get a complete array of necessary vitamins and minerals through our food intake alone, it can be helpful to take a few high-quality supplements. You should never try to get all of your vitamins and minerals by taking supplements. But a high-quality multi-vitamin/multi-mineral supplement as well as a high-quality fiber supplement can be beneficial. Before taking any supplement, we of course recommend that you check with your physician as even "natural" herbal products can have an adverse effect on prescription medicines and medical conditions.

5

MEDITATION AND JOURNALING

An ancient yogi once said the human mind is like a cage filled with a thousand mad monkeys, and the secret to true happiness is your ability to quiet those monkeys. Today you don't have a thousand monkeys. You have five thousand monkeys. Modern technology has given us pagers, cell phones, fax machines and other communication devices with instant text messaging, email and more. As a result of being constantly "in touch," your mind may also be full of everyone *else's* monkeys. Every time someone has an idea, thought, or is simply bored, they can reach you instantly and fill your mind with their thoughts—their monkeys. That's a lot of monkeys.

Much like American housewives in the 1950s who believed that new washing machines, vacuum cleaners and refrigerators would simplify their lives, we have been promised that today's technology will make life simpler and more productive. Unfortunately, this is not the case. This technology simply means that people expect more from us. You are expected to be more available, your work is expected "five minutes ago," and work no longer ends at five o'clock. Work ends when the work is done. But the work is never done. In a global time zone where deadlines exist twenty-four hours a day, we have no time to quiet our minds, no opportunities to get in touch with our inner selves and no opportunities to calm and relax our bodies. This hectic pace promotes stress, anxiety and all the accompanying physical side effects.

For thousands of years man has known the importance of controlling the mind and relaxing the body. The ancients created, then perfected systems to bring quiet from chaos, and passed these disciplines down through the generations. Today medical science is just beginning to understand the connection between the mind and body and its effect on physical health.

Your feelings and thoughts directly influence your body on a chemical level. When you are stressed, angry or scared your body reacts by pumping stress hormones (namely Cortisol) throughout your system. This reaction is known as the "fight or flight" mechanism. When your brain perceives a danger or threat, stress hormones flood the bloodstream, boosting the heart rate and filling the blood with energizing glucose so you can either stand and fight or run away, whichever option will most likely result in the preservation of life. This mechanism also makes blood platelets sticky so that if your body becomes injured, the wound will clot quickly, preventing excessive blood loss. Ideally when the threat subsides, your body returns itself to a normal level of function.

Stop thinking that meditation is anything special. Stop thinking altogether.
-Surya Singer

In the days of the caveman, the fight or flight mechanism kept humans alive. But in today's stressful, over-stimulated world, your body can remain in a perpetual state of strife. This chronic reaction to stress brings on many of negative physical afflictions so prevalent in today's society: high blood pressure, heart disease, poor digestion, weakened immune systems, depression and a host of other ailments.

With all of this in mind, it makes sense to get a handle on your stress triggers, the sources of stress in your life, and the reactions of your mind and body to that stress. Stress reduction and control are equally as important to overall health as are exercise and nutrition. Meditation and positive visualization are some of the most effective stress management tools available, and they are essentially free.

According to a study at Duke University, relaxation techniques like meditation, visualization and yoga, helped people with type II diabetes reduce their blood sugar levels enough to lower their risk of diabetes-related kidney and eye conditions.

Several studies indicate that by simply going to a religious service on a weekly basis—it makes no difference which denomination—increases one's life expectancy by almost seven years. This is about the same number of years you gain by being a non-smoker. The mind is a powerful health management tool and should be included in your daily health and fitness regimen.

We will introduce several different techniques to help you push aside the troubles and pressures of everyday life. Clearly we are each individuals, and what is effective for one may not work for another. The relaxation techniques we will describe are one way, but not the only way to quiet your mind. Find a method that works for you, then practice it on a regular basis—preferably every day. Learning to relax may be more difficult for you than learning Latin. It will take a great deal of discipline to master, but if you are patient and forgiving with yourself, it will be worthwhile. Learning to relax may be the most difficult challenge you face.

Life is like playing a violin in public and learning the instrument as one goes along.
-Samuel Butler

VISUALIZATION

There are many forms of meditation, and visualization is just one of them. As a general rule, Americans find that visualization is the easiest to master. Most of us have been doing it very effectively since we were children. Our son was eight years old and we were having a small party with adults milling around the living room with plates of food and glasses of wine in hand. Suddenly our son burst into to the room, did a spectacular dive roll, came up pointing an imaginary gun, took a few shots at an imaginary bad guy, then trotted from the room. Being the dutiful father, Kent took him aside and said "Son, there were people in there with plates and glasses. What if you had crashed into someone?" Our son replied, "There were *people* in there?" He had created a world in his mind that was so complete and so real that for him, nothing existed outside of it.

That is exactly what we want you to do (with the obvious

exception of the gun fantasy). Start by simply finding a quiet place where there are few distractions. Unplug the telephone, close the door and turn off the television. If it pleases you, softly play some soothing music or simply enjoy the silence. Get into a comfortable position: seated in a comfortable chair, sitting cross-legged on the floor or a pillow or lying flat on your back with arms at your sides.

Breathe slowly, becoming aware of the rhythm that you create with each breath. When you feel yourself begin to relax, picture in your mind the most peaceful, beautiful scene you can imagine. Push aside the outside world and create a quiet, peaceful place within you. You might be lying on a soft towel on a white sand beach in the Caribbean, with gentle ocean breezes caressing your skin. Or see yourself lying in a green field enjoying the fragrance of sweet grass, eucalyptus and wild flowers. Go wherever your heart takes you. The secret: wherever you go, make it *real* for you. Give each of your visualizations detail. Don't be in a hurry to complete the environment, simply enjoy the tour. If you see a tree, don't just see a tree, see an elm tree. Smell the damp soil around the trunk. See the moss on its bark. Start at the top of the tree and work your way through the branches as squirrels scurry along. It is in these details that you will be able to push aside that pressure cooker that you live in each day. In the beginning, even five minutes of uninterrupted thought focused on one of these internal vacations will be difficult. Inevitably, day to day thoughts will pop up—"did I turn off the coffee maker?" "Where did I put my keys when I walked in the door?" Push them gently aside and tell them "Not now."

For years we have trained our minds to multi-task, so we are unused to being single-minded and still. Teaching your mind this new visualization skill will take time, but if you regularly take these mental vacations, the pleasure will draw you back to them and it will no longer feel like an exercise, but a treat to anticipate, savor and enjoy. Visualization is strong medicine, and well worth doing.

All human evil comes from a single cause, man's inability to sit still in a room.
-Blaise Pascal

QUIETING NEGATIVE SELF-TALK

Over the course of a day many of us say negative things to ourselves that we would never say to another person; things we would never allow others to say to us. Some hurtful, demeaning classics are:

- What an idiot
- What a fat pig
- What are you, stupid?
- You are pathetic

This is called negative *self-talk* and we all do it in some form or another. Pull out your own self-talk rolodex and spin through your personal classics—they pop right into your mind, don't they? Negative self-talk can destroy your self-image and self-esteem, or make it impossible to cultivate good feelings about yourself in the first place. While most of us would never accept a coworker, friend or family member saying these things to us, we put up with our own hurtful self-talk every day—maybe even in our dreams!

What most of us need is a way to identify and counter this destructive daily negativity to help us feel better about ourselves. Begin to identify the negative self-talk each time it pops into your head or rolls off your tongue and counter it with a positive affirmation. Mantra meditation is the perfect weapon against negative self-talk and a perfect way to create emotional balance.

Mantra meditation entails creating a mantra (a word or simple phrase) that has significance to you, and repeating it over and over again. Not only does meditation bring awareness to the here and now, it also gives us a chance to practice healthy, positive self-talk. Some healthy new classic mantras might be:

- I feel great
- I look great
- I'm strong
- I have a beautiful soul
- I am loved

The possibilities are endless. Just be sure that they are positive mantras. These mantras also serve another purpose. They become

All of the significant battles are waged within the self.
-Sheldon Kopp

truths. If you say a mantra often enough, you soon believe it. Belief leads to self-truth.

As you say the mantra, aloud or in your head, bring your focus to the words. Become aware of the rhythm they create. Lose yourself in that rhythm. This is more than an exercise in concentration. It is an opportunity to look inside yourself and see the divinity within you. You can combine two or more phrases and repeat them in a series.

Try mantra meditation several times. Give it a fair try. If you find that it does not appeal to you, then try prayer. Prayer is simply another form of meditation. Ten or fifteen minutes of positive prayer can leave you feeling healed and centered. There are many forms of meditation. You may even create your own form of meditation. How you meditate is not important. Just find a form of meditation that works for you and practice it often. Do it every day (see the Day-by day chapter of this book) and you will soon be living your own positive self-truths.

JOURNALING

Journaling is a brief, private time to write about your day. Your journal might be a grade school composition book from the dollar store or an expensive leather-bound tome from a book store. How it looks is unimportant. What is inside is key. Buy a journal and begin to write in it every day. At first, just write about the food you ate.

This can be an eye-opening experience. Those little snacks (4 cookies at 10:00 in the evening) or nibbles (3 homemade brownies in the employee break room during your coffee break) can quickly add up to 1,000 calories over the course of the day! Drinking three 12-ounce cans of Coke® each day adds 420 calories to the bottom line. To burn off that many calories, you'd have to walk about one hour on the treadmill. Don't cheat. Write down everything you put in your mouth. Then look back at your day's food intake and see just how healthy you ate. You will probably be surprised at how many extra snacks and nibbles you indulge in. Your first few weeks of journaling in the Yin Yang Fitness program are only about food because we want you to understand the food choices you make and begin to relate those choices to how your body feels every day.

From simply listing food, you will move into a new phase of journaling in which you will also write down how you felt that day. Were you happy, depressed, tired, energized? Correlate your food intake with your emotional and physical wellbeing. How does the fuel you put into your body affect your emotional state and energy level? At the end of each week, review your journal entries and make some conclusions about the relationship between food and your body.

Your journaling for the second half of Yin Yang Fitness is "freeform journaling" which simply means writing anything and everything about your day. You can make this very creative time and write poetry or music, draw a picture, complain about your boss or mother-in-law, or list your joys and triumphs. Just try not to spend too much time on the negatives--read the inspirational quote for the day if you are having trouble starting.

If you have never written in a journal, it will take some time to get into the habit, so start out simply writing about food and progress from there. In the Day-by-Day chapter, you will find a few open lines at the end of each day. If you don't want to keep a separate journal, you can use this short space to make some daily notes. This is your space; use it however you like.

6

EXERCISE

So, why exercise? If you read the newspaper, watch the news or peruse popular magazines, this question sounds pretty silly. Each day we are bombarded with new studies that show exercise can lower your risk of heart disease and certain types of cancer, lower blood pressure, relieve stress, stengthen bones, elevate your mood, cure depression and jumpstart your libido! Exercise can even help us live longer, more productive, pain-free lives. The list of health benefits goes on. Obviously exercise is good for you. So, if exercise has all these wonderful benefits, why are so few of us doing it?

If you would like to lose fat, exercise is a no-brainer. With all the fad diets and the controversy regarding high carb/low fat or low carb/high fat methods of weight management and scientific-speak about insulin levels and ketosis, it is easy to lose track of the fact that fat loss is actually simple. Burn more calories than you take in and eat moderate-sized portions of good, whole foods (see the nutrition chapter).

Simply do more exercise than you currently do and take in the same number of calories you have been consuming, and you will begin to lose fat. If you burn more calories than you take in, your body must pull from its fat stores for energy, thus depleting your fat surplus.

According to the American Heart Association, twenty-four

percent of Americans age eighteen or older are not active at all. Fifty-four percent of adults get some exercise, but they don't do it regularly or intensely enough to protect their hearts. Only twenty-two percent of American adults get enough leisuretime exercise to achieve cardiopulmonary fitness. With numbers like these it is no wonder more Americans are obese today than at any other time in history. When you combine inactivity with poor food choices in super-size portions it becomes the prescription for a health disaster.

Many of you are exercise refugees because of the way you were taught to exercise. Most of you learned everything you know about exercise from physical education classes in elementary school. At an early age you were taken outside, divided into teams and taught the art of kickball, dodgeball, duck-duck-goose and relay races. If you didn't behave or participate aggressively you were punished with push-ups, chin-ups or laps around the playground--creating a permanent association between exercise, punishment and failure. No doubt this militant approach appealed to some people, but for many of us it alienated us from the simple pleasure of physical activity.

When you combine inactivity with poor food choices in super-size portions it becomes the prescription for a health disaster.

As you got older, teams were chosen for flag football, soccer, basketball and baseball. Status was won and lost with your prowess in these games. Again, punishment for failure was grueling sets of push-ups or laps. Is it any wonder that most of us would rather have root canal than start a new exercise routine?

The secret to success in starting and sticking to an exercise routine is finding something you actually enjoy doing. How do you do that? *Try new things!*

The more you try, the more likely you are to find something you actually like to do. If you like it you will do it. Step outside your comfort zone here. You might be convinced that yoga is too new-age for you, or that you will hate salsa dancing. But you won't find out if you don't try. You just might discover a talent you never knew you had!

Yin Yang fitness is a beginner's guide that will introduce you to contemporary fitness and mind/body exercise, get you more active, broaden your horizons and balance mental and physical activity. As you will see in the Day-by-Day chapter, we blend conventional fitness activities such as weight training and cardiopulmonary exercise (walking, etc.) with the traditional mind/body activities of yoga and pilates.

•You will begin slowly and feel your strength and endurance build.
•You will become aware of the connection between your mind and body.
•Your energy level will soar and you will find yourself wondering how you functioned before without regular exercise.

Our eclectic combination of activity should keep you from becoming bored with exercise. And while we cannot promise you "abs of steel in just six weeks" we would like to help you make the transition from exercise refugee to regular exerciser.

HOW TO USE THE PROGRAM

Reference guides for weight training, yoga and Pilates are included in the following section to help you learn the exercises. Take a few moments to look at the pictures and read the exercise descriptions before your first day on the program. Follow each day for eighty-four days (12 weeks). The program begins at a beginner to moderate level and increases in intensity after each fourteen day period. The exercises change slightly from one fourteen day section to the next, so refer to the new program shown with the fourteen days you are about to begin.

Now, we all know that from time to time life throws us a curve ball--a family emergency, illness or business travel--and by the time we've dealt with it, we've fallen off our routine. At some point this will happen to you. What should you do if you find that a week or two have gone by and you are off the exercise and journaling routine? Don't use this brief hiatus as an excuse to

Fatigue is often caused not by work, but by worry, frustration and resentment. We rarely get tired when we are doing something interesting and exciting.
-Dale Carnegie

quit your healthy new lifestyle. *Start again right away.* Go back to the previous fourteen day program and begin there. Do that program for fourteen days and then continue on as if nothing had happened. Don't be discouraged if you feel sluggish at first--just remember how great you will feel after completing a few days of exercise. Your body's metabolism will remember its efficient rhythms after a few days and will kick back into high gear after a week or so. Don't give up!

WEIGHT TRAINING

You will need:
•One Resist-A-Ball® or other inflated exercise ball
(55mm for most women, 65mm for most men)
•Dumbells
•Comfortable athletic shoes and clothing

Most people have either lifted weights themselves or seen people do it at a gym or on television. Weight training has a number of benefits including increased muscle tone, increased strength, increased bone density (to diminish the advance of osteoporosis), increased metabolism and many more. Weight training is an important part of a comprehensive exercise program. People of any age and fitness level can work out with *some* weight in almost any environment such as home, office, hotel, patio, etc. Yes, almost everyone can and should be doing weight training.

We have chosen dumbells because they are inexpensive, easy to find and buy, portable, and less intimidating for beginners than barbells and machines. The exercises we recommend in this section can be done at home or in a gym with barbells or weight machines if you prefer to work in that environment. Choosing the correct amount of weight will require some experimentation.

It is probably best to get either several dumbells of varying weights or interchangeable-plate dumbells because different muscle groups will be stronger than others and you might need more or less weight to effectively train them. As you continue through the program, we will recommend that you add more weight as you get stronger. You will need dumbells heavy enough that the last few repetitions of your set are very difficult.

Before making a purchase, choose some dumbells and do a test a set of 15 repetitions of one of the exercises. If the weight is correct for your current strength level, then repetition numbers 13, 14 and 15 should be very difficult. You *might* be able to complete a 16th repetition, but you definitely could not get to 17. Before you buy dumbells at a sporting goods store, try several weights with 15 repetitions and see which weight meets your needs.

We have recommended a Resist-A-Ball® instead of a weight bench because the ball is less expensive, easier to store, has many fitness uses, and will force you to work on your core abdominal stability as you train with your weights. In the beginning, it will be a challenge to control the weight during the exercise without falling off the ball, so be careful. Again, it is important to experiment with different weights to make sure that you are using an appropriate weight for your strength and stability level. If the ball proves to be too challenging, you can always switch to a traditional weight bench.

There is no substitute for hard work.
-Thomas Edison

Read the descriptions of the exercises (alphabetically arranged) in the following reference and become familiar with them. Then follow our exercises for each fourteen day segment and all you will have to do is glance at the exercise name and photo to know what to do.

Be sure to move from exercise to exercise quickly with no rest in between. Each day's weight training session is designed to last only fifteen minutes. If you have never worked with weights or a ball before, it may be a good idea to make an appointment with a certified personal trainer to learn how to lift weights with the correct form for your safety.

WEIGHT TRAINING REFERENCE GUIDE

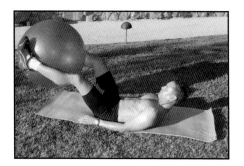

BALL SQUEEZE

Lie down on your back on the mat. Place the ball between your ankles as shown. Raise head and shoulders off mat and tuck chin toward chest. Squeeze the ball between your ankles.

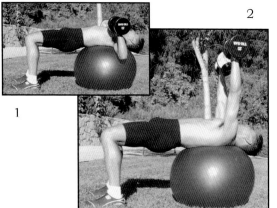

1

2   **BENCH PRESS**

Begin in position 1 with weights directly above shoulders. Press the weights upward until arms are straight. Take one breath, then slowly lower down to starting position and repeat.

BENT OVER ROW

1

Begin in position 1 with weights directly below shoulders. Pull the weights upward until elbows are bent at a 90 degree angle. Take one breath, then slowly lower down to starting position and repeat.

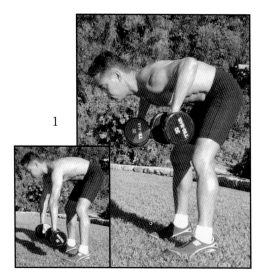

2

WEIGHT TRAINING REFERENCE GUIDE

BICEP CURL

Begin in position 1. With elbows tucked against the sides, pull the weights upward until weights are at shoulder level. Take one breath, then slowly lower down to starting position and repeat.

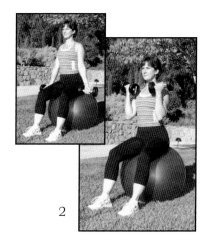

CONCENTRATION CURL

Begin in position 1. With your right elbow braced against your right knee, inhale, then exhale as you bend your elbow and pull the weight upward until it reaches your shoulder. Take one breath, then slowly lower down to starting position. Do your set, then switch arms and repeat.

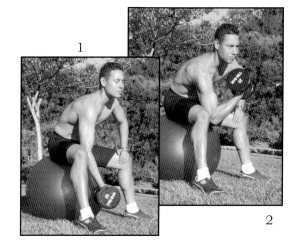

CRUNCH

Begin in position 1 with ball supporting glutes and mid back. Cross arms against your chest. Inhale deeply. Exhale as you do a partial sit-up, isolating your abdominal muscles. Inhale as you lower down to starting position and repeat.

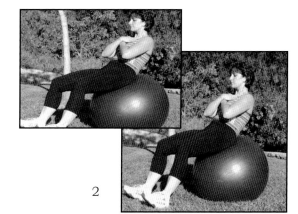

WEIGHT TRAINING REFERENCE GUIDE

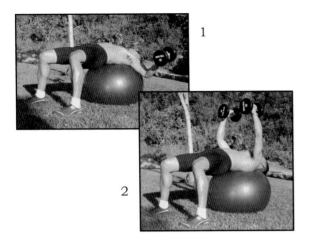

FLY

Begin in position 1 with the ball supporting the lower-mid back. Take a weight in each hand and extend your arms out to your sides with elbows bent as shown. Inhale deeply. Exhale and bring the weights up high over your chest until they almost meet. Inhale and move your arms back to starting position.

LATERAL RAISE

Begin in position 1 seated on the ball. Take a weight in each hand and extend your arms out to your sides with elbows slightly bent as shown. Inhale deeply. Exhale and bring the weights out to the sides. Hold for a two count, then inhale and lower your arms back to starting position.

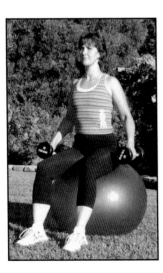
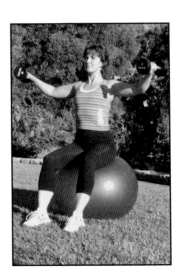

LUNGE

Begin in position 1 with feet together and a weight in each hand. Stand tall. Exhale as you take a long step forward with your left foot. Plant your foot and bend your knee. Be sure that your knee does not extend beyond your toes or you will stress the knee joint. Lower your torso toward the ground. Inhale and push off with your left foot to return to starting position. Switch legs and repeat.

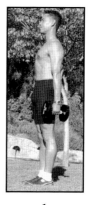

1

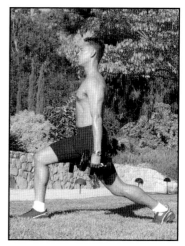

2

SHOULDER PRESS

Begin in position 1 with weights directly above shoulders. Inhale deeply, then exhale as you press the weights upward until arms are straight. Inhale, then slowly lower down to starting position and repeat.

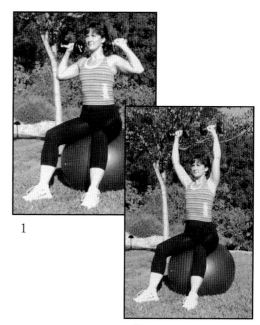

1

2

WEIGHT TRAINING REFERENCE GUIDE

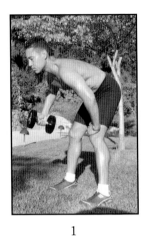

1

SINGLE ARM ROW

Begin in position 1 with weight in one hand directly under shoulder. Inhale deeply, then exhale as you pull the weights upward as far as you can. Inhale, then slowly lower down to starting position and repeat.

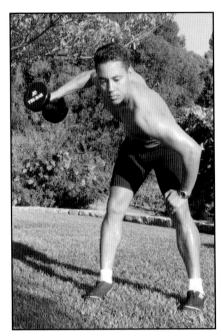

2

1

SQUAT

Begin in position 1 with a weight in each hand and your feet hip-width apart. Inhale deeply as you lower your torso toward the ground until the weights approach knee level. Be sure not to extend your knees out beyond toes. Exhale as you slowly rise back up to starting position.

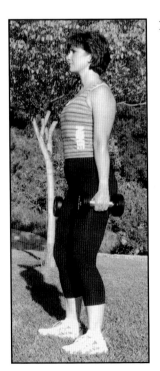

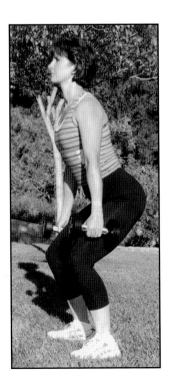

2

WEIGHT TRAINING REFERENCE GUIDE

TOE UP

Begin in position 1 with a weight in each hand and your feet hip-width apart and the front half of each foot on the edge of a step. Inhale deeply as you rise up as high as possible on your toes. Hold in this raised position for three breaths, then on the last exhale, lower toward the ground until you return to starting position.

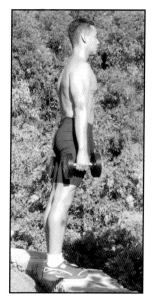 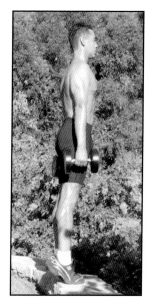

1   2

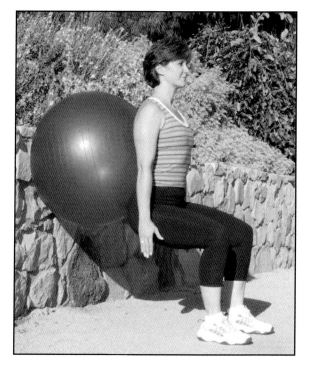

WALL SQUAT

Place the ball behind your mid back and against a wall and press firmly against it with feet about hip-width apart and knees bent as if sitting on a chair. Hold for the suggested number of breaths.

YOGA

You will need:

•A yoga mat
•Comfortable clothing, no socks, no shoes

The exercise known as yoga has been around for more than 5,000 years. Since ancient times, Ayurvedic medicine practitioners have used yoga in combination with food and other therapies to heal patients and help them achieve healthy balance in their lives.

Yoga has countless benefits of a spiritual, physical and mental nature. There are many styles of yoga, from relaxing to athletic. Some yoga asanas (poses) are static stretches or balancing poses which are held while breathing deeply and evenly, in and out through the nose. Some asanas flow smoothly and fluidly from one to the next, creating a dance-like choreography. Regardless of style, even a few minutes each day of relaxing stretches or balancing asanas can yield great progress on the path to a more calm and centered life. Yoga belongs in Yin Yang Fitness, because like everything in this program, it is all about balancing each element with another: cardio with yoga or cardio with weight training. We help you balance rest with work, exercise with meditation, and excellent food choices with "food cheat days" to keep you motivated and encouraged.

If you have never done yoga before, you may want to rent a beginner yoga video and follow along for a session before trying the yoga asanas recommended in Yin Yang Fitness. Watching someone else get into the poses first may help you feel more comfortable as you start this program. Go through the following reference section and read the descriptions next to each photo. Become familiar with the exercises.

YOGA REFERENCE GUIDE

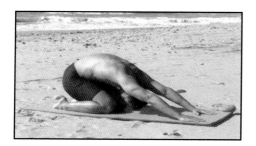

CHILD'S POSE

From hands and knees, sit back on your haunches, buttocks dropping between your heels. Your head drops down toward the floor and arms reach forward as shown. Keeping your hips still, lengthen the spine, walking the hands toward the end of the mat.

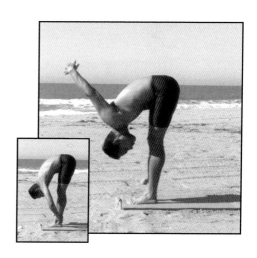

CHEST EXPANSION

From FORWARD FOLD, (inset) bring arms behind body and clasp fingers. Keep a slight bend in the knees to protect the hamstrings. Draw shoulder blades together and widen the chest as you straighten your arms. Look between your legs and rotate your arms so they reach over your head if possible. Imagine that you are clasping an orange between your shoulder blades.

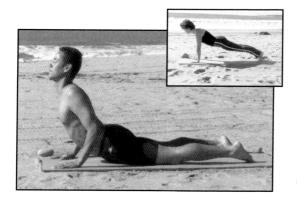

COBRA

From PLANK, (inset) bend elbows, keeping them drawn to sides of body, and sweep chestdown, bringing chest, hips and thigs to mat. Hands should be directly under shoulders. Draw shoulder blades together and widen the chest. Keep arms bent and look straight ahead or slightly upward.

YOGA REFERENCE GUIDE

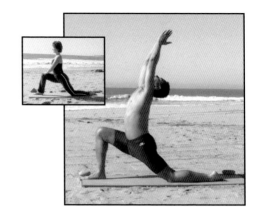

CRESCENT MOON

From RUNNERS LUNGE (inset) draw arms upward and bring palms together overhead. Look up and try to reach further back with your hands. Hold for the suggested number of breaths.

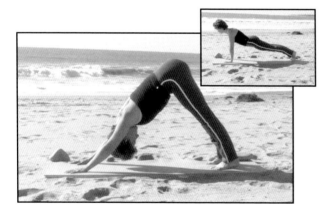

DOWNWARD FACING DOG

From PLANK (inset) push back with arms and bend at the waist. Create an inverted "V" with your body. Try to look at your belly button, encourage your heels to contact the mat and let your head hang between your arms. Hold for the suggested number of breaths.

FORWARD FOLD

From MOUNTAIN pose (inset) draw arms out to the sides as airplane wings, to shoulder level. With a soft bend in the knees, hinge at the hips and swan dive forward with the upper body. Touch the mat if you can, or hold your ankles as shown. Hold for the suggested number of breaths.

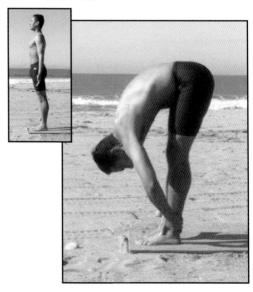

YOGA REFERENCE GUIDE

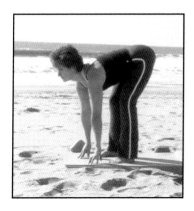

MONKEY

From FORWARD FOLD, inhale and look up, keeping your fingertips on the mat or as close to the mat as possible. Hold for the suggested number of breaths.

MOUNTAIN

With feet about hip-width apart, straighten your spine, draw your shoulder blades together and let your arms hang at sides. Breathe deeply and try to close your eyes. Hold for the suggested number of breaths.

PLANK

Begin on hands and knees, then draw one knee off the floor followed by the other (see picture below left). Be sure that your body is in a straight line, without the glutes pointing up in the air. If this position is too challenging, try the option at right until your strength increases.

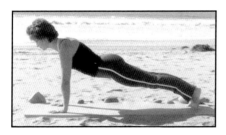

OR

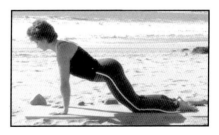

YOGA REFERENCE GUIDE

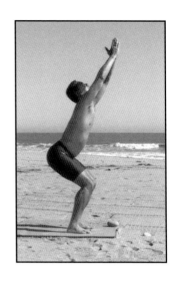

POWERFUL & MIGHTY

With feet about hip-width apart, draw your shoulder blades together and draw both arms overhead as shown. Bend knees and lower torso to create a "lightning bolt" shape in your body. Breathe deeply and hold the pose for the suggested number of breaths.

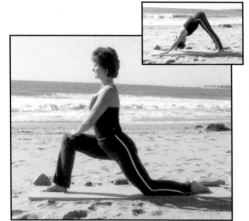

RUNNERS LUNGE

From DOWNWARD FACING DOG (inset) shift your weight forward over your hands and draw the left foot forward between your hands. Rest the right knee on the mat and extend the foot as shown. Bring the hands up to rest on the right knee. Breathe deeply, draw the shoulders back to open the chest and hold the pose for the suggested number of breaths, then switch legs and repeat.

SUNFLOWERS (WARM-UP)

From a standing position, inhale as you raise both arms up high overhead and stretch your abdomen. Begin to exhale and bend your knees, bring your arms down and clasp knees as shown. Inhale and repeat suggested number of times.

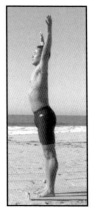

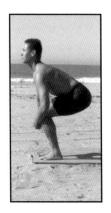

YOGA REFERENCE GUIDE

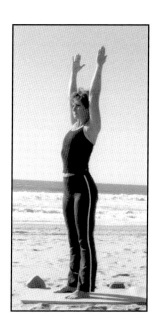

TALL MOUNTAIN

With feet about hip-width apart, draw your shoulder blades together and extend both arms overhead as shown. Lengthen the midsection and try to draw the shoulders back. Breathe deeply and hold the pose for the suggested number of breaths.

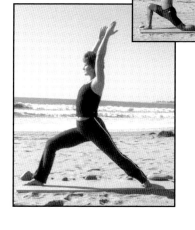

WARRIOR

From CRESCENT MOON (inset) lower both hands to mat and draw weight upward to a balancing standing position so that your forward leg is bent with the knee directly over the ankle. Extend arms overhead and rotate torso forward. Look straight ahead and hold pose for the suggested number of breaths.

PILATES

You will need:

•A yoga mat
•Comfortable clothing, no socks, no shoes

The exercises in the following section are based on the mat exercises created by Joseph Pilates during World War I. A German prison camp internee in England, Pilates developed a system of body conditioning which he taught to his fellow prisoners. While a devastating influenza epidemic swept through Europe killing millions of people, not one prisoner died in the camp where Pilates was teaching his method. He believed that complete health depended upon good circulation and strength of the core abdominal muscles, which he termed the "girdle of strength."

After World War I he emigrated to New York and opened a studio where he trained boxers, dancers and other athletes and performers. His students experienced great gains in strength and explosive power, and the word spread quickly. Pilates classes are now taught in gyms and studios from coast to coast. In addition to mat exercises, he also invented a series of specialized machines that train the core muscle group. While the machines are effective, you need a highly trained and certified Pilates instructor to guide you in their safe use.

The mat exercises are challenging, effective and require no special equipment, can be modified to fit almost any fitness level, and can be performed anywhere you have space to freely move your arms and legs. For Yin Yang Fitness we have selected beginner-to-intermediate modifications for each exercise.

Go through the following reference section and read the descriptions next to each photo to become familiar with the exercises.

PILATES REFERENCE GUIDE

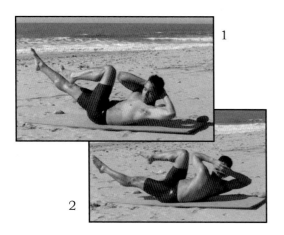

CRISS CROSS

Lie on your back on the mat and lace your fingers behind your head. Bend your left knee and bring it up toward your chest. Extend the right leg out at a 45 degree angle as you twist your torso and draw your right elbow toward the left knee. Reverse and repeat the suggested number of times.

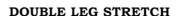

DOUBLE LEG STRETCH

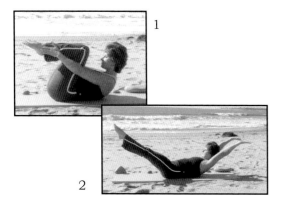

Lie on your back on the mat. Raise your head and shoulders and tuck chin toward chest. Gather your knees to your chest, touching your ankles with your fingers. Inhale as you extend both legs out at a 45 degree angle and draw your arms overhead. Exhale and return to position 1. Repeat the suggested number of times.

THE HUNDRED

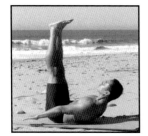

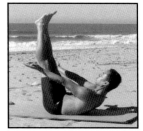

Lie on your back on the mat. Raise your head and shoulders and tuck chin toward chest. Raise your legs as shown. With arms straight and alongside the body, turn the palms upward and inhale the arms upward to knee level, ending at the end of the inhalation. Turn the palms down and exhale to position 1. Repeat the suggested number of times.

PILATES REFERENCE GUIDE

LEG PULLDOWN

From position 1, inhale slowly and raise one leg as shown. Exhale slowly and lower the leg. Repeat the suggested number of times, then switch legs and repeat.

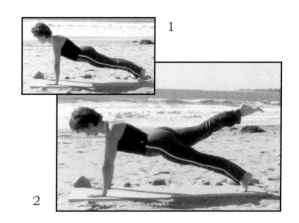

THE SAW

From a seated spread-eagle pose, extend the arms right and left like an airplane and rotate the torso to the right so the fingers of the left hand skim the tops of the toes. Reverse the rotation and repeat the suggested number of times.

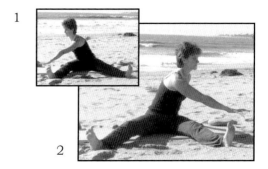

PILATES REFERENCE GUIDE

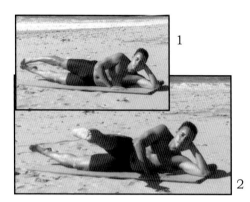

SIDE KICKS

Lie on your side and line up your ankles, knees, hips, shoulders and elbows. Support your head on the lower hand and place the upper hand on the mat as shown. Keep your upper body immobile. Inhale deeply as you slowly move the upper leg forward. Stabilize from the core abdominals. Exhale as you draw the leg back, past the midline of the body as far as you can without moving the upper body. Repeat the suggested number of times, then switch sides and repeat.

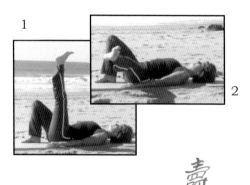

LEG CIRCLES

From position 1, inhale deeply then begin moving the leg out to the left as you begin to exhale. Circle the leg around to the midline of the body and inhale as you draw the leg straight up to position 1, keeping the hips pinned to the mat. Repeat the suggested number of times, then reverse the circle and repeat the suggested number of times.

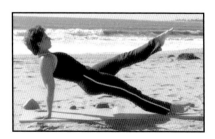

LEG PULL UPS

Begin seated with legs extended in front of you. Place hands on the mat behind the body with fingers pointing away from the body. Raise your hips off the mat until your body is in a straight line. Inhale as you draw the right leg upward as far as possible. Inhale as you draw the leg down again. Repeat the suggested number of times.

PILATES REFERENCE GUIDE

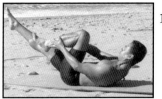 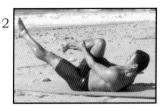

SINGLE LEG STRETCH

Begin lying on your back on the mat with both knees drawn up to chest. Keep head and shoulders on the mat or raise them off the mat as shown. Keep torso stabilized and immobile. Inhale as you extend your right leg out to a 45 degree angle and place both hands on your left ankle as shown in position 1. Exhale and reverse, drawing up the right knee and placing hands on the left ankle as shown in position 2. Repeat the suggested number of times.

SPINE STABILIZER

Begin on hands and knees with the hands directly below the shoulders. Look down at the mat between your hands. Inhale as you extend your right hand and left leg as shown. Hold for a count of three. Exhale as you return to hands and knees. Inhale as you reverse and repeat. Repeat the suggested number of times.

SPINE STRETCH

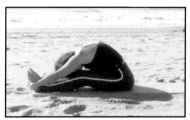

Begin seated with your legs extended in front of you and a slight bend in your knees. Extend your arms, pointing your hands in the direction of your toes. Inhale deeply, then begin to exhale and reach forward slowly toward your toes. Inhale and exhale as you challenge yourself in the stretch and hold it for a few breaths. Repeat the entire process the suggested number of times.

SWIMMING

Lie on your stomach and extend your arms and legs. Tighten your glutes to support your lower back. Inhale deeply and move arms and legs in a gentle swimming motion. Exhale and continue. Continue without stopping for the suggested number of breaths.

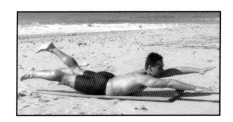

OTHER POSES

FISH

Lie on your back on the mat with legs extended. Place your hands, palms down, beneath your buttocks. Raise the upper body enough to draw the elbows beneath the body as shown, creating an arch in the back. Gently lower the head until the crown of the head touches the mat, or tuck chin to chest and look toward your toes. Hold for the suggested number of breaths.

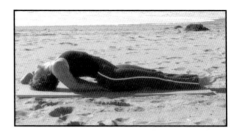

PIGEON

Option A

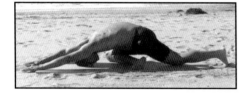

Option A: (For people without knee problems) Begin on hands and knees. Bring your right knee forward and bend the lower half of the leg sideways. Gradually "walk" the left foot backward away from the body until your right calf is beneath the abdomen. Slide the hands forward as far as possible. Hold for the suggested number of breaths, then reverse legs and repeat.

Option B: For people with knee problems. Lie on your back with feet on the mat and knees pointing up. Draw your left knee up toward the chest and cross the left ankle over the right knee (man style). With the left hand, reach through the triangle formed by your left leg and right thigh. Using both hands, clasp the right thigh and draw it gently toward the chest. Relax the shoulders and let the right calf rest on your hands as shown. Hold for the suggested number of breaths, then reverse legs and repeat.

Option B

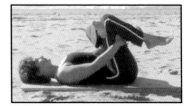

OTHER POSES

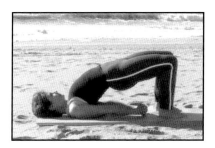

SHOULDER BRIDGE

Lie on your back on the mat with knees pointing up and feet on the mat. Place your hands palms down alongside the body. Inhale as you press your hips upward and create an arch your back. Be sure to rest the weight on your shoulders, not your neck. Hold for the suggested number of breaths, then begin to lower back down beginning at the top of the spine. (If you want more of a challenge, clasp your hands beneath your back and straighten elbows. Walk your shoulder blades closer together.)

SPINE TWIST

Begin seated on the mat with both legs extended in front of you. Draw the left knee up and cross it over the right leg as shown. Straighten the spine and draw the left arm behind the back and place the hand, palm down, as close to the body as possible and straighten the arm. With the right hand, clasp the left knee as shown and look over your left shoulder. Hold for the suggested number of breaths, then reverse and repeat.

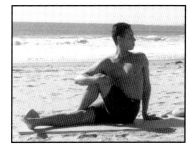

CARDIOPULMONARY (CARDIO) TRAINING
You will need:
•Comfortable, loose-fitting clothing
•Good-fitting, high-quality walking or running shoes
•Optional heartrate monitor

Cardiopulmonary exercise is important to your over-all health because it strengthens the heart, increases lung capacity, creates endurance in the muscles and burns calories. We have chosen walking for Yin Yang Fitness because it is easy, requires no special equipment or gym memberships, you know how to do it, and it gets you outside in nature breathing fresh air. You might prefer to substitute a different form of cardio work such as step classes, cardio kick-boxing, bicycling with your family, salsa dancing, hiking, swimming, etc. Do something you like, because that will help you to continue doing it. Staying with it is what is important.

In the Day-by-Day fitness section we will mention keeping yourself at a "target heart-rate" for a certain number of minutes. This means that by exercising at a designated percentage of your maximum heart rate you are effectively training your cardiopulmonary system. You should never attempt to train for any length of time at your maximum heart rate because not only would that be incredibly uncomfortable, it would be very dangerous. We know this sounds confusing, but let us explain:

First you must establish your approximate maximum heart rate. Begin with the number 220. Deduct your age, and that is your approximate maximum heart rate. To find your target heart rate, multiply your *maximum heart rate* by the suggested percentage. For example, Bob is a 30 year-old man. To establish his approximate *target heart rate* of 65-75% of his maximum heart rate, he would do this:

220 - 30 = 190 (approximate maximum heartrate)
190 x .65 = 123.5 heart beats per minute
Next,
190 x .75 = 142.5 heart beats per minute

With these two calculations in hand, Bob now knows that for the first fourteen days of Yin Yang Fitness, he would want to walk at a pace that would keep his heart beating at a rate of between 123 and 142 beats per minute.

The most reliable and convenient method to monitor your heartrate while exercising is with a heartrate monitor available at most sporting goods stores and ranging in cost and quality. You can also take your own pulse during exercise by placing your finger (not your thumb) on your carotid artery at the front of your neck or finding your pulse at your wrist and counting the number of beats in ten seconds and multiplying by six.

The mind/body way to find your approximate heart rate during exercise is the *perceived exertion test.* Ask yourself, on a scale of one to ten, "how do I feel right now?" One would be "I'm asleep" and ten would be "I am exercising so hard that I think I'm going to die!" You would like to exercise at a level that you would consider to be between six and eight on that scale. (For example, at *nine* you would be unable to talk and exercise at the same time. At *four* you might feel like you could do this level of activity all day with no problem.) You can use the perceived exertion test in conjunction with your heartrate monitor to get in touch with how you are feeling at any time during your exercise. This method helps you to tune in to the signals your body is sending.

7

DAY-BY-DAY

You are about to take your first step on the path to better health. As with any journey, the path may be long and challenging. Ahead there may be potholes and rocks, but the path is also surrounded by beauty and self-discovery and the rewards are many. The most difficult challenge is to continue walking down that path. Enjoy the journey. Be in the moment. Read the quotations and words of wisdom on each day's page. Share them with others in your life. Revel in the pleasure when someone notices that you look calmer, thinner, or more confident. They *will* notice.

As you begin Yin Yang Fitness, notice that each seventh day is a day of complete rest; you might wish to begin on the correct day so that your day of rest from the program falls on a day off work or school so you can fully relax. Rest is important.

When you have completed the program, we believe that you will feel better, stronger and more in control of your life and health. But what then, you ask. The beauty of Yin Yang Fitness is that during this twelve weeks you will still be living your real life. You will still be eating real food, with some healthy changes. You will not have been on an overly restricted "diet" or drinking shakes at mealtime. Yin Yang fitness is a lifestyle that can be sustained over the long haul.

You will have modified your lifestyle to make room for the new you. All you have to do is continue with healthy routines.

Your body could go on with this program indefinitely and be balanced and healthy. Hopefully, you will like the way you feel. If yoga works for you, find a yoga class in your community and sign up. If you are enjoying cooking healthy recipes, take cooking classes. Stay active, give your body enough of what it needs, but not too much. The path continues, and now you can choose its direction.

Should you have a question about the program or need clarification, you can email us at our website: www.mylifefitness.com or www.amberwoodpress.com. We will do our best to answer every email we receive. We wish you the best.

Namaste, (the divine in us bows to the divine in you)

Kent and Maria

WEIGHT TRAINING FOR THE FIRST FOURTEEN DAYS (15 minute session)

Complete one set of 15 reps of each exercise for the first fourteen days as directed.

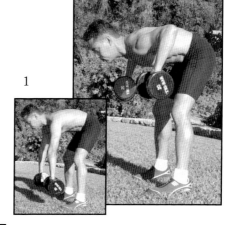

BENT OVER ROW

(15 REPS)

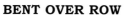

BICEP CURL

(15 REPS)

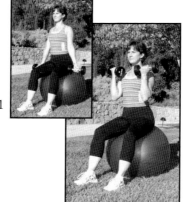

LUNGES

(15 REPS)

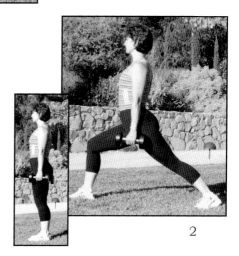

WEIGHT TRAINING FOR THE FIRST FOURTEEN DAYS (15 minute session)
Complete one set of 15 reps of each exercise for the first fourteen days as directed.

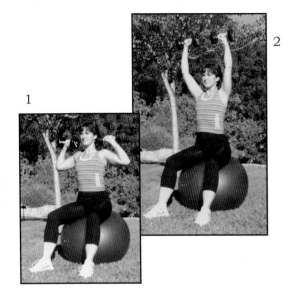

SHOULDER PRESS
(15 REPS)

WALL SQUATS
(HOLD FOR 45-60 SECONDS)

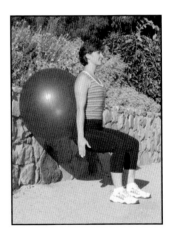

BENCH PRESS
(15 REPS)

WEIGHT TRAINING FOR THE FIRST FOURTEEN DAYS (15 minute session)

Complete one set of 15 reps of each exercise for the first fourteen days as directed.

TOE UPS

(15 REPS)

壽

CRUNCHES

(15 REPS)

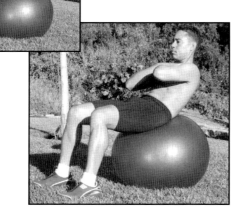

YOGA FOR THE FIRST FOURTEEN DAYS

Cycle through this routine continuously for 10-15 minutes as directed.

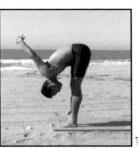

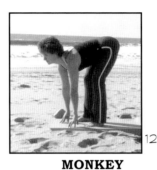

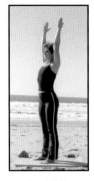

13

12

11

MONKEY
(3 BREATHS)

TALL MOUNTAIN
(3 BREATHS)

CHEST EXPANSION
(3 BREATHS)

END
HERE

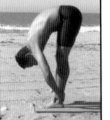

10

FORWARD FOLD
(3 BREATHS)

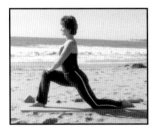

9

RUNNER'S LUNGE
(3 BREATHS EACH LEG)

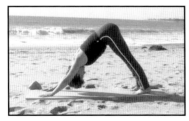

8

**DOWNWARD FACING
DOG**
(3 BREATHS)

7

COBRA
(3 BREATHS)

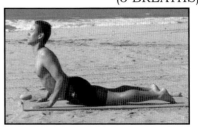

YOGA FOR THE FIRST FOURTEEN DAYS

Cycle through this routine continuously for 10-15 minutes as directed.

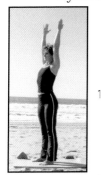

SUNFLOWERS

(5 BREATHS)

1

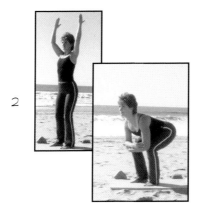

2

TALL MOUNTAIN

(3 BREATHS)

BEGIN

HERE

3

FORWARD FOLD

(3 BREATHS)

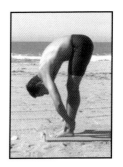

4

CHEST EXPANSION

(3 BREATHS)

6

5

PLANK

(1BREATH)

MONKEY

(3 BREATHS)

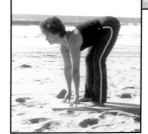

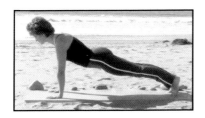

EXERCISE DAY-BY-DAY

Day One

☐   Five minutes of visualization

☐   Cardio: Do thirty minutes of brisk walking at 65%-75% of your maximum heart rate on a flat course

☐   Weights: Do the suggested weight program for fifteen minutes moving from task to task with no rest in between

☐   Five minutes of journaling about the food you ate and how you feel.

Notes for the day.....

The beginning is the most important part of the work.
-Plato

_____

_____

_____

_____

_____

_____

Day Two

☐   Five minutes of visualization

☐   Cardio: Do thirty minutes of brisk walking at 65%-75% of your maximum heart rate on a flat course

☐   Yoga: Do the suggested yoga program for fifteen minutes moving from asana to asana with no rest in between

When we see men of worth, we should think of equaling them; when we see men of contrary character, we should turn inwards and examine our- selves.
-Confucious

☐   Five minutes of journaling about the food you ate and how you feel.

Notes for the day.....

_____

_____

_____

_____

_____

_____

_____

Day Three

☐ Five minutes of visualization

☐ Cardio: Do thirty minutes of brisk walking at 65%-75% of your maximum heart rate on a flat course

☐ Weights: Do the suggested weight program for fifteen minutes moving from task to task with no rest in between

☐ Five minutes of journaling about the food you ate and how you feel.

Tell me, I'll forget. Show me, I may remember. But involve me and I'll understand.
-Chinese Proverb

Notes for the day.....

_____

_____

_____

_____

_____

_____

Day Four

☐ Five minutes of visualization

☐ Cardio: Do thirty minutes of brisk walking at 65%-75% of your maximum heart rate on a flat course

☐ Yoga: Do the suggested yoga program for fifteen minutes moving from asana to asana with no rest in between

☐ Five minutes of journaling about the food you ate and how you feel.

Genius is nothing more or less than childhood recovered by will, a childhood now equipped for self-expression with an adult's capacities.
-Charles Baudelaire

Notes for the day.....

_____

_____

_____

_____

_____

_____

Day Five

☐ Five minutes of visualization

☐ Cardio: Do thirty minutes of brisk walking at 65%-75% of your maximum heart rate on a flat course

☐ Weights: Do the suggested weight program for fifteen minutes moving from task to task with no rest in between

☐ Five minutes of journaling about the food you ate and how you feel.

Notes for the day.....

A man only learns in two ways, one by reading, and the other by associating with smarter people.
-Will Rogers

_____

_____

_____

_____

_____

_____

Day Six

☐   Five minutes of visualization

☐   Yoga: Do the suggested yoga program for fifteen minutes moving from asana to asana with no rest in between

☐   Five minutes of writing in your food journal.

Anyone who stops learning is old, whether twenty or eighty. Anyone who keeps learning today is young. The greatest thing in life is to keep your mind young.
-Henry Ford

Notes for the day.....

_____

_____

_____

_____

_____

_____

Day Seven

☐   Five minutes of visualization

☐   This is a no exercise day and a cheat day for nutrition. Just try to eat healthy portions of foods that you love. Perhaps give yourself a special treat.

☐   Five minutes of writing in your journal about how you feel at the end of this week.

The world is our school for spiritual discovery.
-Paul Brunton

Notes for the day.....

_____

_____

_____

_____

_____

_____

Day Eight

☐ Five minutes of visualization

☐ Cardio: Do thirty minutes of brisk walking at 65%-75% of your maximum heart rate on a flat course

☐ Weights: Do the suggested weight program for fifteen minutes moving from task to task with no rest in between

☐ Five minutes of journaling about the food you ate and how you feel.

There are costs and risks to a program of action, but they are far less than the long range risks and costs of comfortable inaction.
-John F. Kennedy

Notes for the day.....

_____

_____

_____

_____

_____

_____

_____

Day Nine

☐ Five minutes of visualization

☐ Cardio: Do thirty minutes of brisk walking at 65%-75% of your maximum heart rate on a flat course

☐ Yoga: Do the suggested yoga program for fifteen minutes moving from asana to asana with no rest in between

☐ Five minutes of journaling about the food you ate and how you feel.

It is easier to go down a hill than up, but the view is from the top.
-Arnold Bennett

Notes for the day.....

_____

_____

_____

_____

_____

_____

Day Ten

☐ Five minutes of visualization

☐ Cardio: Do thirty minutes of brisk walking at 65%-75% of your maximum heart rate on a flat course

☐ Weights: Do the suggested weight program for fifteen minutes moving from task to task with no rest in between

☐ Five minutes of journaling about the food you ate and how you feel.

Only those who will risk going too far can possibly find out how far one can go.
-T.S. Elliot

Notes for the day.....

_____

_____

_____

_____

_____

_____

Day Eleven

☐   Five minutes of visualization

☐   Cardio: Do thirty minutes of brisk walking at 65%-75% of your maximum heart rate on a flat course

☐   Yoga: Do the suggested yoga program for fifteen minutes moving from asana to asana with no rest in between

☐   Five minutes of journaling about the food you ate and how you feel.

Notes for the day.....

In all human affairs there are efforts, and there are results, and the strength of the effort is the measure of the result.
-James Allen

_____

_____

_____

_____

_____

Day Twelve

☐   Five minutes of visualization

☐   Cardio: Do thirty minutes of brisk walking at 65%-75% of
     your maximum heart rate on a flat course

☐   Weights: Do the suggested weight program for fifteen
     minutes moving from task to task with no rest in between

☐   Five minutes of journaling about the food you ate and how
     you feel.

Let me not pray to be sheltered from dangers but to be fearless in facing them. Let me not beg for the stilling of my pain but for the heart to conquer it.
-Tagore

Notes for the day.....

_____

_____

_____

_____

_____

_____

Day Thirteen

☐   Five minutes of visualization

☐   Yoga: Do the suggested yoga program for fifteen minutes moving from asana to asana with no rest in between

☐   Five minutes of journaling about the food you ate and how you feel.

Notes for the day.....

Carpenters bend wood; fletchers bend arrows; wise men fashion themselves.
-Buddha

_____

_____

_____

_____

_____

_____

Day Fourteen

☐ Five minutes of visualization

☐ This is a no exercise day and a cheat day for nutrition. Just try to eat healthy portions of foods that you love. Perhaps give yourself a special treat.

☐ Five minutes of writing in your journal about how you feel at the end of this week.

Congratulations! You have completed the first two weeks of Yin Yang Fitness. In order to challenge your stronger body, your exercises will change slightly for the next two weeks.

*In the long run you hit only what you aim at. Therefore, though you should fail immediately, you had better aim at something high.
-Henry David Thoreau*

Notes for the day.....

_____

_____

_____

_____

_____

_____

_____

WEIGHT TRAINING FOR THE SECOND FOURTEEN DAYS (15 minute session)

Increase the weight of your dumbells and decrease the number of repetitions to 12 of each exercise for the second fourteen days as directed.

BENT OVER ROW
(12 REPS)

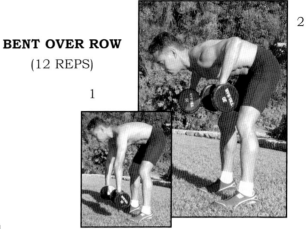

BICEP CURL
(12 REPS)

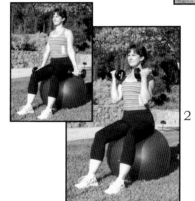

LUNGES
(12 REPS)

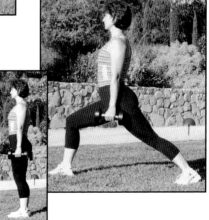

WEIGHT TRAINING FOR THE SECOND FOURTEEN DAYS (15 minute session)

Increase the weight of your dumbells and decrease the number of repetitions to 12 of each exercise for the second fourteen days as directed.

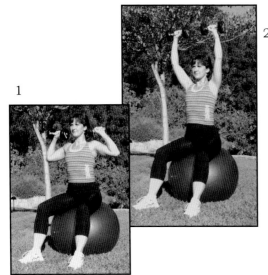

SHOULDER PRESS

(12 REPS)

WALL SQUATS

(HOLD FOR 45-60 SECONDS)

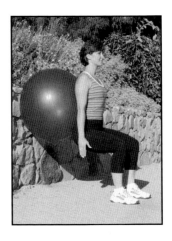

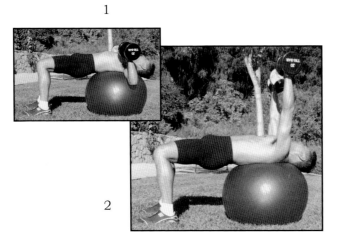

BENCH PRESS

(12 REPS)

WEIGHT TRAINING FOR THE SECOND FOURTEEN DAYS (15 minute session)

Increase the weight of your dumbells and decrease the number of repetitions to 12 of each exercise for the second fourteen days as directed.

TOE UPS
(12 REPS)

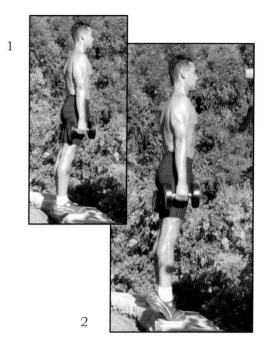

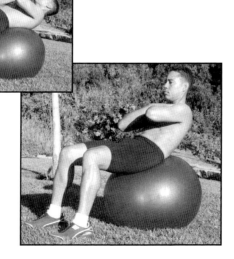

CRUNCHES
(12 REPS)

YOGA FOR THE SECOND FOURTEEN DAYS

Cycle through this routine continuously for 15 minutes as directed.

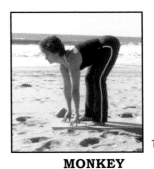

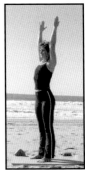

15

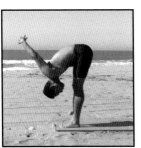

14

MONKEY

(3 BREATHS)

13

TALL MOUNTAIN

(3 BREATHS)

CHEST EXPANSION

(3 BREATHS)

END
HERE

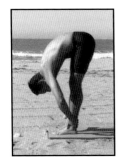

12

FORWARD FOLD

(3 BREATHS)

11

WARRIOR I

(3 BREATHS)

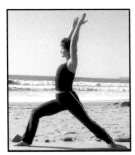

10

CRESCENT MOON

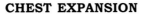

(3 BREATHS)

9

RUNNER'S LUNGE

(3 BREATHS EACH LEG)

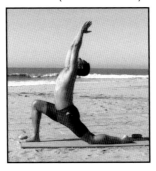

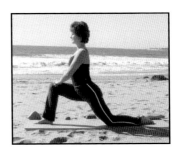

YOGA FOR THE SECOND FOURTEEN DAYS

Cycle through this routine continuously for15 minutes as directed.

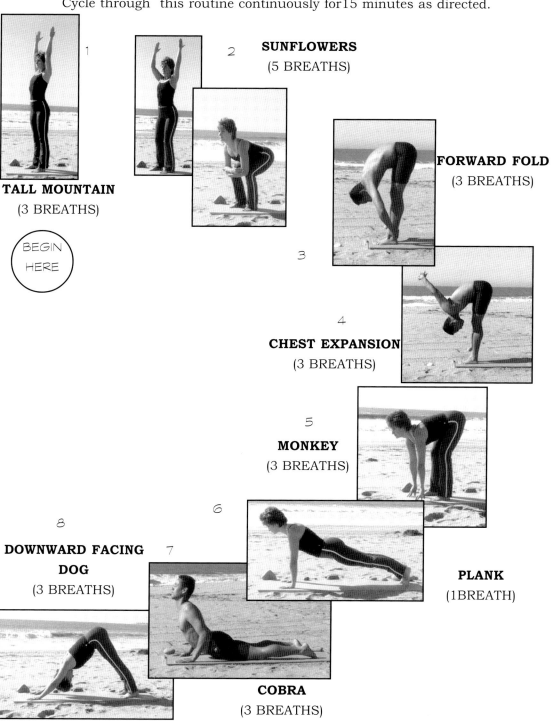

1

2 **SUNFLOWERS**
(5 BREATHS)

FORWARD FOLD
(3 BREATHS)

TALL MOUNTAIN
(3 BREATHS)

BEGIN HERE

3

4

CHEST EXPANSION
(3 BREATHS)

5

MONKEY
(3 BREATHS)

6

8

**DOWNWARD FACING
DOG**
(3 BREATHS)

7

PLANK
(1BREATH)

COBRA
(3 BREATHS)

Day Fifteen

☐ Five minutes of visualization

☐ Cardio: Do thirty minutes of brisk walking or jogging at 65% - 75% of your maximum heart rate on a course that varies from flat to moderately hilly

☐ Weights: Do the suggested weight program for fifteen minutes moving from task to task with no rest in between

☐ Five minutes of journaling about the food you ate and how you feel.

I am a great believer in luck, and I find that the harder I work, the more I have of it.
-Thomas Jefferson

Notes for the day.....

_____

_____

_____

_____

_____

_____

Day Sixteen

☐ Five minutes of visualization

☐ Cardio: Do thirty minutes of brisk walking or jogging at 65%-75% of your maximum heart rate on a course that varies from flat to moderately hilly

☐ Yoga: Do the suggested yoga program for fifteen minutes moving from asana to asana with no rest in between

☐ Five minutes of journaling about the food you ate and how you feel.

*Look within.
Within is the
fountain of good,
and it will ever
bubble up, if thou
wilt ever dig.
-Marcus Aurelius*

Notes for the day.....

_____

_____

_____

_____

_____

_____

Day Seventeen

☐ Five minutes of visualization

☐ Cardio: Do thirty minutes of brisk walking or jogging at 65%-75% of your maximum heart rate on a course that varies from flat to moderately hilly

☐ Weights: Do the suggested weight program for fifteen minutes moving from task to task with no rest in between

☐ Five minutes of journaling about the food you ate and how you feel.

Notes for the day.....

_____

_____

_____

_____

_____

_____

All labor that uplifts humanity has dignity and importance and should be undertaken with painstaking excellence.
-Martin Luther King, Jr.

Day Eighteen

☐ Five minutes of visualization

☐ Cardio: Do thirty minutes of brisk walking at 65%-75% of your maximum heart rate on a course that varies from flat to moderately hilly

☐ Yoga: Do the suggested yoga program for fifteen minutes moving from asana to asana with no rest in between

☐ Five minutes of journaling about the food you ate and how you feel.

I have often been asked what I thought was the secret of Buddha's smile. It is - it can only be - that he smiles at himself for searching all those years for what he already possessed.
-Paul Brunton

Notes for the day.....

_____

_____

_____

_____

_____

_____

Day Nineteen

☐   Five minutes of visualization

☐   Cardio: Do thirty minutes of brisk walking at 65%-75% of
     your maximum heart rate on a course that varies from flat
     to moderately hilly

☐   Weights: Do the suggested weight program for fifteen
     minutes moving from task to task with no rest in be-
     tween

☐   Five minutes of journaling about the food you ate and how
     you feel.

*Self-esteem is the
reputation we
acquire with
ourselves.*
-Nathaniel Branden

Notes for the day.....

_____

_____

_____

_____

_____

_____

Day Twenty

☐   Five minutes of visualization

☐   Yoga: Do the suggested yoga program for fifteen minutes
        moving from asana to asana with no rest in between

☐   Five minutes of journaling about the food you ate and
        how you feel.

*Always bear in
mind that your
own resolution to
succeed is more
important than
any other one
thing.
-Abraham Lincoln*

Notes for the day.....

_____

_____

_____

_____

_____

_____

_____

Day Twenty-one

☐   Five minutes of visualization

☐   This is a no exercise day and a cheat day for nutrition.
     Just try to eat healthy portions of foods that you love.
     Perhaps give yourself a special treat.

☐   Five minutes of writing in your journal about how you feel
     at the end of this week.

*We look backward
too much and we
look forward too
much; thus we
miss the only
eternity of which
we can be abso-
lutely sure--the
eternal present, for
it is always now.
-William Phelps*

Notes for the day.....

_____

_____

_____

_____

_____

_____

Day Twenty-two

☐   Five minutes of visualization

☐   Cardio: Do thirty minutes of brisk walking or jogging at
      65% - 75% of your maximum heart rate on a course that
      varies from flat to moderately hilly

☐   Weights: Do the suggested weight program for fifteen
      minutes moving from task to task with no rest in between

*Hold yourself
responsible for a
higher standard
than anyone else
expects of you.
Never excuse
yourself.
-Henry Ward
Beecher*

☐   Five minutes of journaling about the food you ate and how
      you feel.

Notes for the day.....

_____

_____

_____

_____

_____

_____

_____

Day Twenty-three

☐ Five minutes of visualization

☐ Cardio: Do thirty minutes of brisk walking or jogging at 65%-75% of your maximum heart rate on a course that varies from flat to moderately hilly

☐ Yoga: Do the suggested yoga program for fifteen minutes moving from asana to asana with no rest in between

☐ Five minutes of journaling about the food you ate and how you feel.

Notes for the day.....

_____

_____

_____

_____

_____

_____

People are always blaming their circumstances for what they are. I don't believe in circumstances. The people who get on in this world are the people who get up and look for the circumstances they want, and, if they can't find them, make them.
-George Bernard Shaw

Day Twenty-four

☐   Five minutes of visualization

☐   Cardio: Do thirty minutes of brisk walking or jogging at 65%-75% of your maximum heart rate on a course that varies from flat to moderately hilly

☐   Weights: Do the suggested weight program for fifteen minutes moving from task to task with no rest in between

☐   Five minutes of journaling about the food you ate and how you feel.

Fear always springs from ignorance.
-Ralph Waldo Emerson

Notes for the day.....

_____

_____

_____

_____

_____

_____

Day Twenty-five

☐   Five minutes of visualization

☐   Cardio: Do thirty minutes of brisk walking at 65%-75% of your maximum heart rate on a course that varies from flat to moderately hilly

☐   Yoga: Do the suggested yoga program for fifteen minutes moving from asana to asana with no rest in between

☐   Five minutes of journaling about the food you ate and how you feel.

Notes for the day.....

Self-knowledge and self-improvement are very difficult for most people. It usually needs great courage and long struggle.
-Abraham Maslow

_____

_____

_____

_____

_____

_____

Day Twenty-six

☐   Five minutes of visualization

☐   Cardio: Do thirty minutes of brisk walking at 65%-75% of your maximum heart rate on a course that varies from flat to moderately hilly

☐   Weights: Do the suggested weight program for fifteen minutes moving from task to task with no rest in between

☐   Five minutes of journaling about the food you ate and how you feel.

As the physically weak man can make himself strong by careful and patient training, so the man of weak thoughts can make them strong by exercising himself in right thinking.
-James Allen

Notes for the day.....

_____

_____

_____

_____

_____

_____

Day Twenty-seven

☐ Five minutes of visualization

☐ Yoga: Do the suggested yoga program for fifteen minutes moving from asana to asana with no rest in between

☐ Five minutes of journaling about the food you ate and how you feel.

Notes for the day.....

_____

_____

_____

_____

_____

_____

Happiness doesn't depend on what we have, but it does depend on how we feel towards what we have. We can be happy with little and miserable with much.
-W.D. Hoard

Day Twenty-eight

☐   Five minutes of visualization

☐   This is a no exercise day and a cheat day for nutrition. Just try to eat healthy portions of foods that you love. Perhaps give yourself a special treat.

☐   Five minutes of writing in your journal about how you feel at the end of this week.

In every block of marble I see a statue as plain as though it stood before me, shaped and perfect in attitude and action. I have only to hew away the rough walls that imprison the lovely apparition to reveal it to other eyes as mine see it.
-Michelangelo

Congratulations! You have completed the second two weeks of Yin Yang Fitness. In order to challenge your stronger body, your exercises will change slightly for the next two weeks.

Notes for the day.....

_____

_____

_____

_____

_____

_____

WEIGHT TRAINING FOR THE THIRD FOURTEEN DAYS (15 minute session)

Complete one set of 12 reps of each exercise. Then, switch to a heavier weight and do a second set of 10 reps of each exercise. Remember to move from exercise to exercise as quickly as possible with no rest in between.

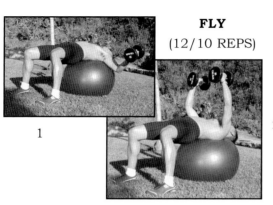

FLY
(12/10 REPS)

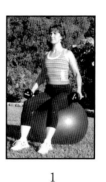

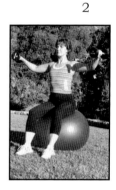

LATERAL RAISES
(12/10 REPS)

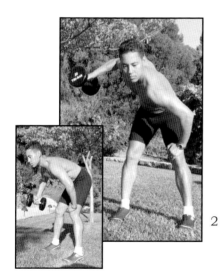

**SINGLE ARM
ROWS**
(12/10 REPS)

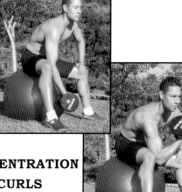

**CONCENTRATION
CURLS**
(12/10 REPS)

WEIGHT TRAINING FOR THE THIRD FOURTEEN DAYS (15 minute session)

Complete one set of 12 reps of each exercise. Then, switch to a heavier weight and do a second set of 10 reps of each exercise. Remember to move from exercise to exercise as quickly as possible with no rest in between.

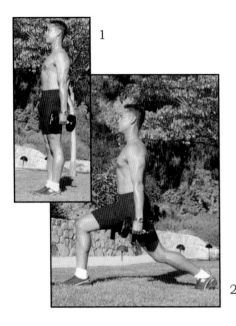

LUNGES
(12/10 REPS)

SQUATS
(12/10 REPS)

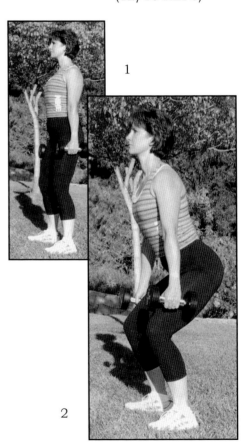

BALL SQUEEZES
(12/10 REPS)

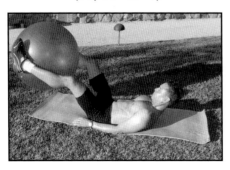

PILATES FOR THE THIRD FOURTEEN DAYS (15 minute session)

Flow from exercise to exercise doing the designated number of repetitions.

THE HUNDRED

(10 REPS)

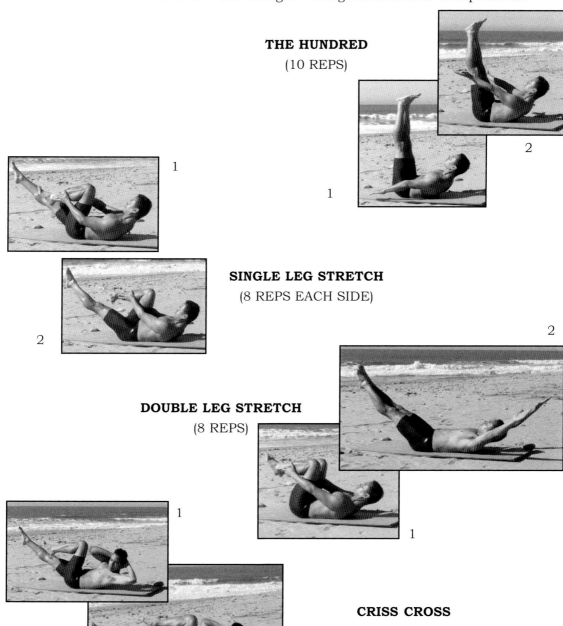

SINGLE LEG STRETCH

(8 REPS EACH SIDE)

DOUBLE LEG STRETCH

(8 REPS)

CRISS CROSS

(10 REPS ALTERNATING SIDES)

PILATES FOR THE THIRD FOURTEEN DAYS (15 minute session)

Flow from exercise to exercise doing the designated number of repetitions.

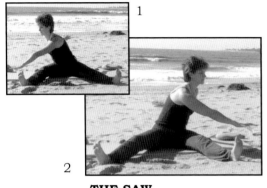

THE SAW

(10 REPS EACH SIDE)

SIDE KICKS

(8 REPS EACH SIDE)

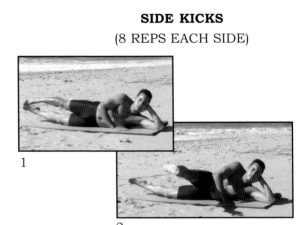

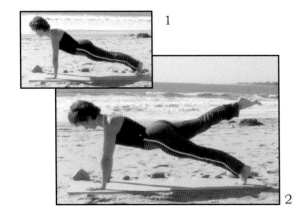

LEG PULL DOWNS

(8 REPS EACH SIDE)

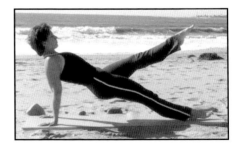

LEG PULL UPS

(4 REPS EACH SIDE)

Day Twenty-nine

☐   Ten minutes of visualization

☐   Cardio: Do thirty to forty-five minutes of brisk walking or jogging at 75%-85% of your maximum heart rate on a hilly course

☐   Weights: Do the suggested weight program for fifteen minutes moving from task to task with no rest in between

☐   Ten minutes of journaling about the food you ate and how you feel.

The future belongs to those who believe in the beauty of their dreams.
-Eleanor Roosevelt

Notes for the day.....

_____

_____

_____

_____

_____

_____

Day Thirty

☐   Ten minutes of visualization

☐   Cardio: Do thirty to forty-five minutes of brisk walking or jogging at 75%-85% of your maximum heart rate on a hilly course

☐   Pilates: Do the suggested Pilates exercises for fifteen minutes with no rest in between

☐   Ten minutes of journaling about the food you ate and how you feel.

*To know oneself,
one should assert
oneself.
-Albert Camus*

Notes for the day.....

_____

_____

_____

_____

_____

_____

_____

Day Thirty-one

☐   Ten minutes of visualization

☐   Cardio: Do thirty to forty-five minutes of brisk walking or
     jogging at 75%-85% of your maximum heart rate on a hilly
     course

☐   Weights: Do the suggested weight program for fifteen
     minutes moving from task to task with no rest in between

☐   Five minutes of journaling about the food you ate and how
     you feel.

*If you refuse to
accept anything
but the best out of
life, you very often
get it.
-Somerset Maughn*

Notes for the day.....

_____

_____

_____

_____

_____

_____

Day Thirty-two

☐   Ten minutes of visualization

☐   Cardio: Do thirty to forty-five minutes of brisk walking at
       75% - 85% of your maximum heart rate on a hilly course

☐   Pilates: Do the suggested Pilates exercises for fifteen
       minutes with no rest in between.

☐   Ten minutes of journaling about the food you ate and how
       you feel.

*Thinking is the
hardest work
there is, which is
the probable
reason why so
few people
engage in it.
-Henry Ford*

Notes for the day.....

_____

_____

_____

_____

_____

_____

Day Thirty-three

☐ Ten minutes of visualization

☐ Cardio: Do thirty to forty-five minutes of brisk walking at 75%-85% of your maximum heart rate on a hilly course

☐ Weights: Do the suggested weight program for fifteen minutes moving from task to task with no rest in between

☐ Ten minutes of journaling about the food you ate and how you feel.

Notes for the day.....

Nurture your mind with great thoughts. To believe in the heroic makes heroes.
-Benjamin Disraeli

_____

_____

_____

_____

_____

Day Thirty-four

☐   Ten minutes of visualization

☐   Pilates: Do the suggested Pilates exercises for fifteen minutes with no rest in between

☐   Ten minutes of journaling about the food you ate and how you feel.

Whatever you do or dream you can do- begin it. Boldness has a genius and power and magic in it. -Johann Goethe

Notes for the day.....

_____

_____

_____

_____

_____

_____

Day Thirty-five

☐   Ten minutes of visualization

☐   This is a no exercise day and a cheat day for nutrition.
      Just try to eat healthy portions of foods that you love.
      Perhaps give yourself a special treat.

☐   Ten minutes of writing in your journal about how you feel
      at the end of this week.

*The happiness of
your life depends
on the quality of
your thoughts.
-Marcus Aurelius*

Notes for the day.....

_____

_____

_____

_____

_____

_____

Day Thirty-six

☐   Ten minutes of visualization

☐   Cardio: Do thirty to forty-five minutes of brisk walking or jogging at 75%-85% of your maximum heart rate on a hilly course

☐   Weights: Do the suggested weight program for fifteen minutes moving from task to task with no rest in between

☐   Ten minutes of journaling about the food you ate and how you feel.

Strength doesn't come from physical capacity. It comes from indomitable will.
-Mahatma Gandhi

Notes for the day.....

_____

_____

_____

_____

_____

_____

Day Thirty-seven

☐   Ten minutes of visualization

☐   Cardio: Do thirty to forty-five minutes of brisk walking or
     jogging at 75%-85% of your maximum heart rate on a
     hilly course

☐   Pilates: Do the suggested Pilates exercises for fifteen
     minutes with no rest in between

☐   Ten minutes of journaling about the food you ate and how
     you feel.

Notes for the day.....

*Within your own
house dwells the
treasure of joy; so
why do you go
begging from door
to door?
-Sufi Saying*

_____

_____

_____

_____

_____

_____

Day Thirty-eight

☐   Ten minutes of visualization

☐   Cardio: Do thirty to forty-five minutes of brisk walking or jogging at 75%-85% of your maximum heart rate on a hilly course

☐   Weights: Do the suggested weight program for fifteen minutes moving from task to task with no rest in between

No one can make you feel inferior without your consent.
-Eleanor Roosevelt

☐   Five minutes of journaling about the food you ate and how you feel.

Notes for the day.....

_____

_____

_____

_____

_____

_____

Day Thirty-nine

☐   Ten minutes of visualization

☐   Cardio: Do thirty to forty-five minutes of brisk walking at
     75% - 85% of your maximum heart rate on a hilly course

☐   Pilates: Do the suggested Pilates exercises for fifteen
     minutes with no rest in between

☐   Ten minutes of journaling about the food you ate and how
     you feel.

*Laughter is the
jam on the toast of
life. It adds flavor,
keeps it from being
too dry, and
makes it easier to
swallow.
-Diane Johnson*

Notes for the day.....

_____

_____

_____

_____

_____

_____

Day Forty

☐   Ten minutes of visualization

☐   Cardio: Do thirty to forty-five minutes of brisk walking at 75%-85% of your maximum heart rate on a hilly course

☐   Weights: Do the suggested weight program for fifteen minutes moving from task to task with no rest in between

☐   Ten minutes of journaling about the food you ate and how you feel.

Courage is grace under pressure.
-Ernest Hemingway

Notes for the day.....

_____

_____

_____

_____

_____

_____

Day Forty-one

☐ Ten minutes of visualization

☐ Pilates: Do the suggested Pilates exercises for fifteen minutes with no rest in between

☐ Ten minutes of journaling about the food you ate and how you feel.

Notes for the day.....

The mind is the great leveler of all things; human thought is the process by which human ends are ultimately answered.
-Daniel Webster

_____

_____

_____

_____

_____

_____

Day Forty-two

☐   Ten minutes of visualization

☐   This is a no exercise day and a cheat day for nutrition. Just try to eat healthy portions of foods that you love. Perhaps give yourself a special treat.

Nothing in the world can take the place of persistence. Talent will not; nothing is more common than unsuccessful men with talent. Genius will not; unrewarded genius is almost a proverb. Education will not; the world is full of educated derelicts. Persistence and determination alone are omnipotent.
-Calvin Coolidge

☐   Ten minutes of writing in your journal about how you feel at the end of this week.

Congratulations! You have completed the third two weeks of Yin Yang Fitness. In order to challenge your stronger body, your exercises will change slightly for the next two weeks.

Notes for the day.....

———————————————————————

———————————————————————

———————————————————————

———————————————————————

———————————————————————

———————————————————————

———————————————————————

WEIGHT TRAINING FOR THE FOURTH FOURTEEN DAYS (15 minute session)

Using the weight you used for the second set of reps in the last fourteen day segment, complete one set of 10 reps of each exercise. Then, switch to a heavier weight and do a second set of 8 reps of each exercise. Remember to move from exercise to exercise as quickly as possible with no rest in between.

FLY
(10/8 REPS)

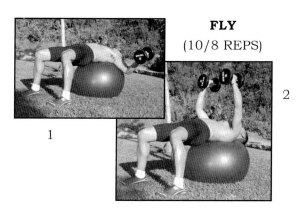

LATERAL RAISES
(10/8 REPS)

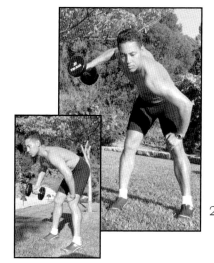

**SINGLE ARM
ROWS**
(10/8 REPS)

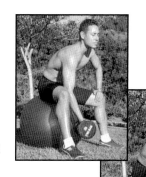

**CONCENTRATION
CURLS**
(10/8 REPS)

WEIGHT TRAINING FOR THE FOURTH FOURTEEN DAYS (15 minute session)

Using the weight you used for the second set of reps in the last fourteen day segment, complete one set of 10 reps of each exercise. Then, switch to a heavier weight and do a second set of 8 reps of each exercise. Remember to move from exercise to exercise as quickly as possible with no rest in between.

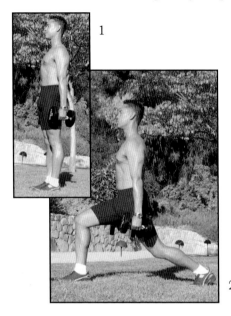

LUNGES

(10/8 REPS)

SQUATS

(10/8 REPS)

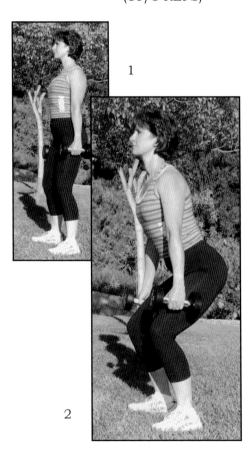

BALL SQUEEZES

(10/8 REPS)

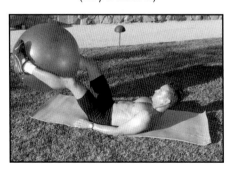

PILATES FOR THE FOURTH FOURTEEN DAYS (15-20 minute session)

Flow from exercise to exercise doing the designated number of repetitions.

THE HUNDRED
(10 REPS)

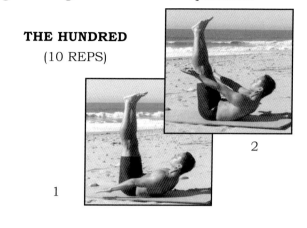

2

1

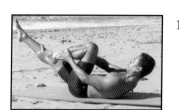

1

SINGLE LEG STRETCH
(8 REPS EACH SIDE)

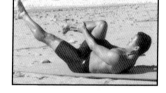

2

2

DOUBLE LEG STRETCH
(8 REPS)

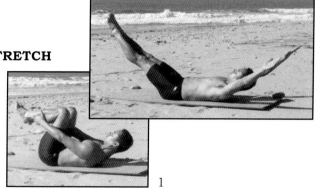

1

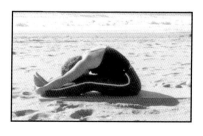

SPINE STRETCH
(HOLD FOR 5 BREATHS)

PILATES FOR THE FOURTH FOURTEEN DAYS (15-20 minute session)

Flow from exercise to exercise doing the designated number of repetitions.

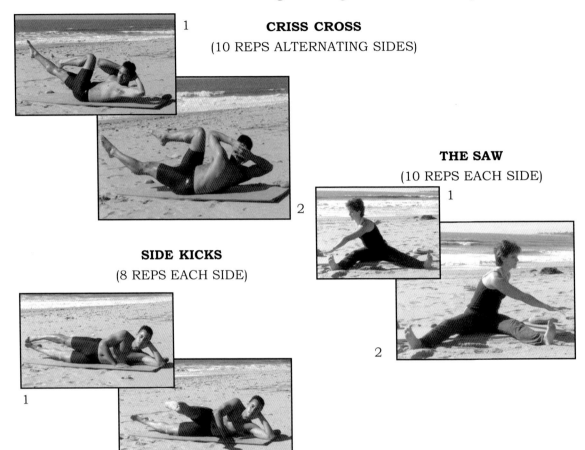

CRISS CROSS

(10 REPS ALTERNATING SIDES)

THE SAW

(10 REPS EACH SIDE)

SIDE KICKS

(8 REPS EACH SIDE)

SWIMMING

(8 BREATHS)

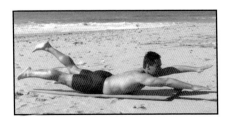

PILATES FOR THE FOURTH FOURTEEN DAYS (15-20 minute session)

Flow from exercise to exercise doing the designated number of repetitions.

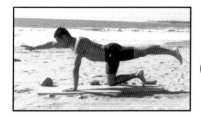

SPINE STABILIZER
(8 MOVEMENTS ALTERNATING SIDES)

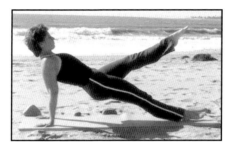

LEG PULL UPS
(4 REPS EACH SIDE)

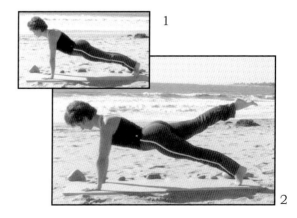

LEG PULL DOWNS
(8 REPS EACH SIDE)

Day Forty-three

☐ Ten minutes of visualization

☐ Cardio: Do thirty to forty-five minutes of alternating between one minute of walking or jogging at a brisk pace, and walking or jogging at a moderate pace on a flat course

☐ Weights: Do the suggested weight program for fifteen minutes moving from task to task with no rest in between

☐ Ten minutes of freeform journaling.

There is no security in life, only opportunity.
-Mark Twain

Notes for the day.....

_____

_____

_____

_____

_____

_____

Day Forty-four

☐   Ten minutes of visualization

☐   Cardio: Do thirty to forty-five minutes of alternating
      between one minute of walking or jogging at a brisk pace,
      and walking or jogging at a moderate pace on a flat course

☐   Pilates: Do the suggested Pilates exercises for fifteen
      minutes with no rest in between

☐   Ten minutes of freeform journaling.

*Life can be
understood
backwards; but it
must be lived
forwards.
-Soren
Kierkegaard*

Notes for the day.....

_____

_____

_____

_____

_____

_____

Day Forty-five

☐   Ten minutes of visualization

☐   Cardio: Do thirty to forty-five minutes of alternating
     between one minute of walking or jogging at a brisk pace,
     and walking or jogging at a moderate pace on a flat course

☐   Weights: Do the suggested weight program for fifteen
     minutes moving from task to task with no rest in be-
     tween

☐   Ten minutes of freeform journaling.

*Not knowing how
near the truth is,
people seek it far
away, what a pity!
They are like him
who, in the midst of
water, cries in thirst
so imploringly.
-Hakuin*

Notes for the day.....

_____

_____

_____

_____

_____

_____

Day Forty-six

☐ Ten minutes of visualization

☐ Cardio: Do thirty to forty-five minutes of alternating between one minute of walking or jogging at a brisk pace, and
walking or jogging at a moderate pace on a flat course

☐ Pilates: Do the suggested Pilates exercises for fifteen
minutes with no rest in between

☐ Ten minutes of freeform journaling.

*Too many people
spend money
they haven't
earned, to buy
things they don't
want, to impress
people they don't
like.
-Will Rogers*

Notes for the day.....

_____

_____

_____

_____

_____

_____

Day Forty-seven

☐   Ten minutes of visualization

☐   Cardio: Do thirty to forty-five minutes of alternating between one minute of walking or jogging at a brisk pace, and walking or jogging at a moderate pace on a flat course

☐   Weights: Do the suggested weight program for fifteen minutes moving from task to task with no rest in between

☐   Ten minutes of freeform journaling.

The great secret of success is to go through life as a man who never gets used to failing.
-Albert Schweitzer

Notes for the day.....

_____

_____

_____

_____

_____

Day Forty-eight

☐   Ten minutes of visualization

☐   Pilates: Do the suggested Pilates exercises for fifteen
     minutes with no rest in between

☐   Ten minutes of freeform journaling.

*Every minute you
are angry, you
lose sixty seconds
of happiness.
-Ralph Waldo
Emerson*

Notes for the day.....

_____

_____

_____

_____

_____

_____

Day Forty-nine

☐ Ten minutes of visualization

☐ This is a no exercise day and a cheat day for nutrition.
Just try to eat healthy portions of foods that you love.
Perhaps give yourself a special treat.

☐ Ten minutes of freeform journaling.

Notes for the day.....

_____

_____

_____

_____

_____

_____

*Nothing would be
done at all if a
man waited until
he could do it so
well that no one
could find fault
with it.
-Cardinal Newman*

Day Fifty

☐   Ten minutes of visualization

☐   Cardio: Do thirty to forty-five minutes of alternating be-
      tween one minute of walking or jogging at a brisk pace,
      and walking or jogging at a moderate pace on a flat course

☐   Weights: Do the suggested weight program for fifteen
      minutes moving from task to task with no rest in between

One of the sim-   ☐   Ten minutes of freeform journaling.
plest things about
all the facts of life
is that to get
where you want
to go, you must   *Notes for the day.....*
keep on keeping
on.
-Norman Vincent   ———————————————————————————
Peale

———————————————————————————

———————————————————————————

———————————————————————————

———————————————————————————

———————————————————————————

Day Fifty-one

☐   Ten minutes of visualization

☐   Cardio: Do thirty to forty-five minutes of alternating between one minute of walking or jogging at a brisk pace, and
walking or jogging at a moderate pace on a flat course

☐   Pilates: Do the suggested Pilates exercises for fifteen
minutes with no rest in between

☐   Ten minutes of freeform journaling.

*What a wonderful
life I've had! I only
wish I'd realized it
sooner.
-Collette*

Notes for the day.....

_____

_____

_____

_____

_____

_____

Day Fifty-two

☐   Ten minutes of visualization

☐   Cardio: Do thirty to forty-five minutes of alternating be-
     tween one minute of walking or jogging at a brisk pace, and
     walking or jogging at a moderate pace on a flat course

☐   Weights: Do the suggested weight program for fifteen
     minutes moving from task to task with no rest in between

☐   Ten minutes of freeform journaling.

*Ask and it shall
be given unto
you. Seek and ye
shall find.
-Luke 11:9*

Notes for the day.....

_____

_____

_____

_____

_____

_____

_____

Day Fifty-three

☐   Ten minutes of visualization

☐   Cardio: Do thirty to forty-five minutes of alternating between one minute of walking or jogging at a brisk pace,
and walking or jogging at a moderate pace on a flat course

☐   Pilates: Do the suggested Pilates exercises for fifteen
minutes with no rest in between

☐   Ten minutes of freeform journaling.

Notes for the day.....

_____

_____

_____

_____

_____

_____

I have learned this at least by my experiment: that if one advances confidently in the direction of his dreams, and endeavors to live the life which he has imagined, he will meet with success unexpected in common hours.
-Henry David Thoreau

Day Fifty-four

☐ Ten minutes of visualization

☐ Cardio: Do thirty to forty-five minutes of alternating between one minute of walking or jogging at a brisk pace, and
walking or jogging at a moderate pace on a flat course

☐ Weights: Do the suggested weight program for fifteen
minutes moving from task to task with no rest in between

☐ Ten minutes of freeform journaling.

*If you must begin
then go all the
way, because if
you begin and
quit, the unfin-
ished business
you have left
behind begins to
haunt you all the
time.
-Chogyam
Trungpa*

Notes for the day.....

_____

_____

_____

_____

_____

_____

_____

Day Fifty-five

☐   Ten minutes of visualization

☐   Pilates: Do the suggested Pilates exercises for fifteen
     minutes with no rest in between

☐   Ten minutes of freeform journaling.

Notes for the day.....

_____

_____

_____

_____

_____

_____

*Thousands of
people have talent.
I might as well
congratulate you
for having eyes in
your head. The
one and only thing
that counts is: do
you have staying
power?
-Noel Coward*

Day Fifty-six

☐   Ten minutes of visualization

☐   This is a no exercise day and a cheat day for nutrition. Just try to eat healthy portions of foods that you love. Perhaps give yourself a special treat.

☐   Ten minutes of freeform journaling.

One word frees us of all the weight and pain of life: that word is love.
-Sophocles

Congratulations! You have completed the fourth two weeks of Yin Yang Fitness. In order to challenge your stronger body, your exercises will change for the next two weeks.

Notes for the day.....

_____

_____

_____

_____

_____

_____

_____

WEIGHT TRAINING FOR THE FIFTH FOURTEEN DAYS (15 minute session)
Using the weight you used for the second set of reps in the last fourteen day segment, complete one set of 6 reps of each exercise, but this time move in slow motion (a slow count to 14 as you raise the weights and another slow count to 14 as you lower the weights). Remember to move from exercise to exercise as quickly as possible with no rest in between.

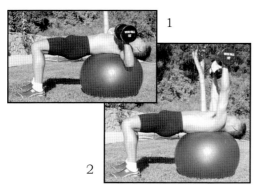

BENCH PRESS
(6 SLOW-MOTION REPS)

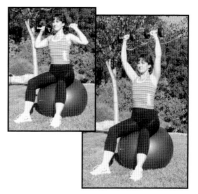

SHOULDER PRESS
(6 SLOW-MOTION REPS)

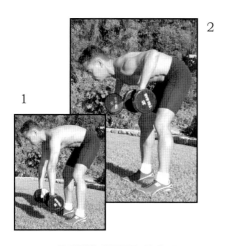

BENT OVER ROW
(6 SLOW-MOTION REPS)

BICEP CURL
(6 SLOW-MOTION REPS)

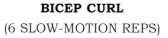
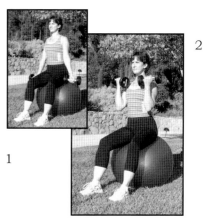

WEIGHT TRAINING FOR THE FIFTH FOURTEEN DAYS (15 minute session)

Using the weight you used for the second set of reps in the last fourteen day segment, complete one set of 6 reps of each exercise, but this time move in slow motion (a slow count to 14 as you raise the weights and another slow count to 14 as you lower the weights). Remember to move from exercise to exercise as quickly as possible with no rest in between.

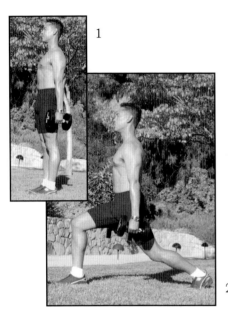

LUNGES
(6 SLOWMOTION REPS)

WALL SQUATS
(HOLD FOR 45-60 SECONDS)

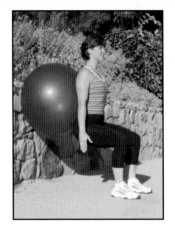

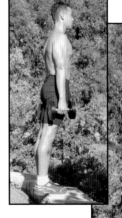

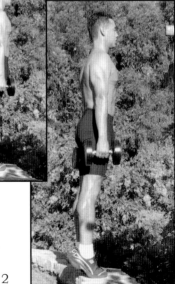

TOE UPS
(6 SLOW-MOTION
REPS)

YOGA/PILATES BLEND FOR THE FIFTH FOURTEEN DAYS
(15-20 minute session)

Flow from exercise to exercise doing the designated number of repetitions.

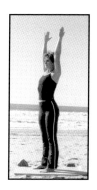

TALL MOUNTAIN

(3 BREATHS)

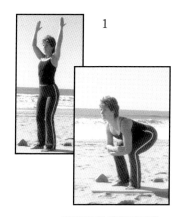

SUNFLOWERS

(5 BREATHS)

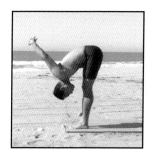

CHEST EXPANSION

(3 BREATHS)

PLANK
(1BREATH)

COBRA
(3 BREATHS)

DOWNWARD FACING DOG
(3 BREATHS)

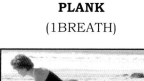
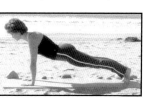
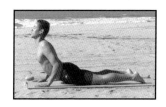

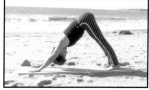

COMPLETE THE ABOVE SERIES (PLANK, COBRA, DOWN DOG)
THREE TIMES BEFORE MOVING ON TO SPINE STABILIZER.

YOGA/PILATES BLEND FOR THE FIFTH FOURTEEN DAYS
(15-20 minute session)

Flow from exercise to exercise doing the designated number of repetitions.

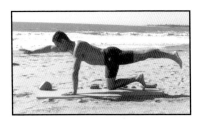

SPINE STABILIZER

(8 MOVEMENTS ALTERNATING SIDES)

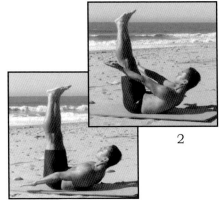

2

1

THE HUNDRED

(10 REPS)

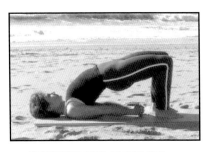

SHOULDER BRIDGE

(5 BREATHS)

2

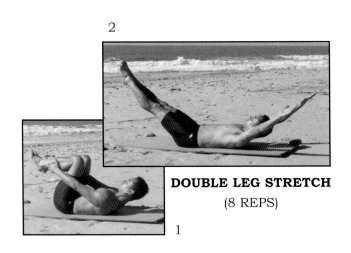

DOUBLE LEG STRETCH

(8 REPS)

1

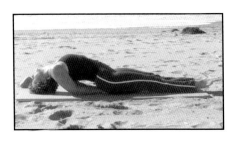

FISH POSE

(5 BREATHS)

YOGA/PILATES BLEND FOR THE FIFTH FOURTEEN DAYS
(15-20 minute session)

Flow from exercise to exercise doing the designated number of repetitions.

LEG CIRCLES
(8 REPS EACH LEG)

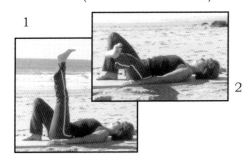

SPINE TWIST
(5 BREATHS)

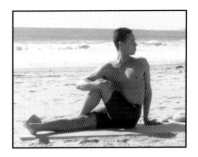

SIDE KICKS
(8 REPS EACH SIDE)

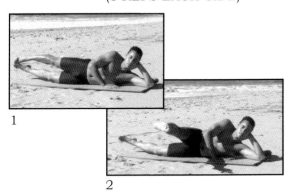

PIGEON POSE
(5 BREATHS)

Option A

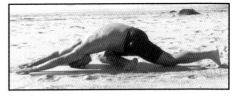

Option B

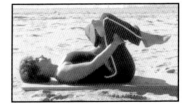

YOGA/PILATES BLEND FOR THE FIFTH FOURTEEN DAYS
(15-20 minute session)
Flow from exercise to exercise doing the designated number of repetitions.

SWIMMING
(8 BREATHS)

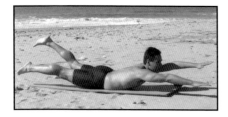

CHILD'S POSE
(5 BREATHS)

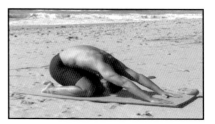

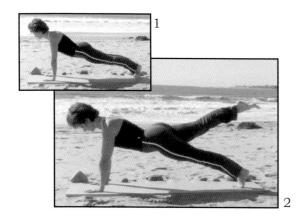

LEG PULL DOWNS
(8 REPS EACH SIDE)

CHILD'S POSE
(5 BREATHS)

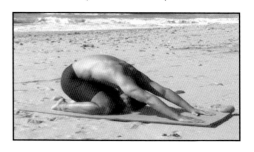

Day Fifty-seven

☐   Fifteen minutes of meditation

☐   Cardio: Do thirty to forty-five minutes of alternating between one minute of walking or jogging at a brisk pace, and walking or jogging at a moderate pace on a course that varies from flat to moderately hilly

☐   Weights: Do the suggested weight program with slow-motion repetitions for twenty minutes moving from task to task with no rest in between

☐   Fifteen minutes of freeform journaling.

It's not the size of the dog in a fight, it's the size of the fight in the dog.
-Kit Raymond

Notes for the day.....

_____

_____

_____

_____

_____

_____

Day Fifty-eight

☐ Fifteen minutes of meditation

☐ Cardio: Do thirty to forty-five minutes of alternating between one minute of walking or jogging at a brisk pace, and
walking or jogging at a moderate pace on a course that
varies from flat to moderately hilly

☐ Yoga/Pilates Blend: Do the suggested blend exercises for
fifteen minutes with no rest in between

The best thing   ☐ Fifteen minutes of freeform journaling.
about the future
is that it comes
only one day at a
time.
-Abraham Lincoln   *Notes for the day.....*

_____

_____

_____

_____

_____

_____

Day Fifty-nine

☐ Fifteen minutes of meditation

☐ Cardio: Do thirty to forty-five minutes of alternating between one minute of walking or jogging at a brisk pace, and
walking or jogging at a moderate pace on a course that
varies from flat to moderately hilly

☐ Weights: Do the suggested weight program with slow-
motion repetitions for fifteen minutes moving from task to
task with no rest in between

☐ Fifteen minutes of freeform journaling.

*Love truth, but
pardon error.*
-Voltaire

Notes for the day.....

_____

_____

_____

_____

_____

_____

Day Sixty

☐   Fifteen minutes of meditation

☐   Cardio: Do thirty to forty-five minutes of alternating be-
     tween one minute of walking or jogging at a brisk pace, and
     walking or jogging at a moderate pace on a course that
     varies from flat to moderately hilly

☐   Yoga/Pilates Blend: Do the suggested blend exercises for
     fifteen minutes with no rest in between

The highest yoga   ☐   Fifteen minutes of freeform journaling.
is the control of
the mind.
-Srimad
Bhagavatam   *Notes for the day.....*

_____

_____

_____

_____

_____

_____

Day Sixty-one

☐   Fifteen minutes of meditation

☐   Cardio: Do thirty to forty-five minutes of alternating
       between one minute of walking or jogging at a brisk pace,
       and walking or jogging at a moderate pace on a course
       that varies from flat to moderately hilly

☐   Weights: Do the suggested weight program with slow
       motion repetitions for fifteen minutes moving from task
       to task with no rest in between

☐   Fifteen minutes of freeform journaling.

*The man of virtue
makes the
difficulty to be
overcome his first
business, and
success only a
subsequent
consideration.
-Confucius*

Notes for the day.....

_____

_____

_____

_____

_____

Day Sixty-two

☐ Fifteen minutes of meditation

☐ Yoga/Pilates Blend: Do the suggested blend exercises for fifteen minutes with no rest in between

☐ Fifteen minutes of freeform journaling.

Come out of the circle of time, and into the circle of love.
-Rumi

Notes for the day.....

_____

_____

_____

_____

_____

_____

Day Sixty-three

☐ Fifteen minutes of meditation

☐ This is a no exercise day and a cheat day for nutrition. Just try to eat healthy portions of foods that you love. Perhaps give yourself a special treat.

☐ Fifteen minutes of freeform journaling.

The best portion of a good man's life-- his little, nameless, unremembered acts of kindness and of love.
-William Wordsworth

Notes for the day.....

_____

_____

_____

_____

_____

_____

Day Sixty-four

☐   Fifteen minutes of meditation

☐   Cardio: Do thirty to forty-five minutes of alternating between one minute of walking or jogging at a brisk pace, and
walking or jogging at a moderate pace on a course that
varies from flat to moderately hilly

☐   Weights: Do the suggested weight program with slow-
motion repetitions for fifteen minutes moving from task to
task with no rest in between

*There is no royal
road to anything.
One thing at a time,
and all things in
succession. That
which grows slowly
endures.
-Joshua Holland*

☐   Fifteen minutes of freeform journaling.

Notes for the day.....

_____

_____

_____

_____

_____

_____

Day Sixty-five

☐ Fifteen minutes of meditation

☐ Cardio: Do thirty to forty-five minutes of alternating between one minute of walking or jogging at a brisk pace, and walking or jogging at a moderate pace on a course that varies from flat to moderately hilly

☐ Yoga/Pilates Blend: Do the suggested blend exercises for fifteen minutes with no rest in between

☐ Fifteen minutes of freeform journaling.

Notes for the day.....

Great works are perfomed not by strength but by perseverence.
-Samuel Johnson

_____

_____

_____

_____

_____

_____

Day Sixty-six

☐ Fifteen minutes of meditation

☐ Cardio: Do thirty to forty-five minutes of alternating between one minute of walking or jogging at a brisk pace, and walking or jogging at a moderate pace on a course that varies from flat to moderately hilly

☐ Weights: Do the suggested weight program with slow-motion repetitions for fifteen minutes moving from task to task with no rest in between

What then is your duty? What the day demands.
-Johann Goethe

☐ Fifteen minutes of freeform journaling.

Notes for the day.....

_____

_____

_____

_____

_____

_____

Day Sixty-seven

☐ Fifteen minutes of meditation

☐ Cardio: Do thirty to forty-five minutes of alternating between one minute of walking or jogging at a brisk pace,
and walking or jogging at a moderate pace on a course that
varies from flat to moderately hilly

☐ Yoga/Pilates Blend: Do the suggested blend exercises for
fifteen minutes with no rest in between

☐ Fifteen minutes of freeform journaling.

*Those who know
do not speak and
those who speak
do not know.
-Lao-tzu*

Notes for the day.....

_____

_____

_____

_____

_____

_____

Day Sixty-eight

☐ Fifteen minutes of meditation

☐ Cardio: Do thirty to forty-five minutes of alternating between one minute of walking or jogging at a brisk pace, and
walking or jogging at a moderate pace on a course that
varies from flat to moderately hilly

☐ Weights: Do the suggested weight program with slow
motion repetitions for fifteen minutes moving from task to
task with no rest in between

Your imagination is your preview of life's coming attractions.
-Albert Einstein

☐ Fifteen minutes of freeform journaling.

Notes for the day.....

_____

_____

_____

_____

_____

_____

Day Sixty-nine

☐   Fifteen minutes of meditation

☐   Yoga/Pilates Blend: Do the suggested blend exercises for
fifteen minutes with no rest in between

☐   Fifteen minutes of freeform journaling.

Notes for the day.....

When we quit thinking primarily about ourselves and our own self-preservation, we undergo a truly heroic trasformation of consciousness.
-Joseph Campbell

_____

_____

_____

_____

_____

_____

Day Seventy

☐ Fifteen minutes of meditation

☐ This is a no exercise day and a cheat day for nutrition. Just try to eat healthy portions of foods that you love. Perhaps give yourself a special treat.

☐ Fifteen minutes of freeform journaling.

The true meaning of life is to plant trees, under whose shade you do not expect to sit.
-Nelson Henderson

Congratulations! You have completed the fifth two weeks of Yin Yang Fitness.

Notes for the day.....

_____

_____

_____

_____

_____

_____

WEIGHT TRAINING FOR THE SIXTH FOURTEEN DAYS (15 minute session)
If you can, add some the weight to what you used in the last fourteen day segment. Complete one set of 6 reps of each exercise in slow motion (a slow count to 14 as you raise the weights and another slow count to 14 as you lower the weights). Remember to move from exercise to exercise as quickly as possible with no rest in between.

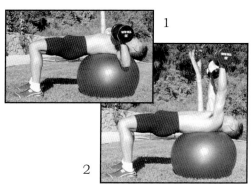

BENCH PRESS
(6SLOW-MOTION REPS)

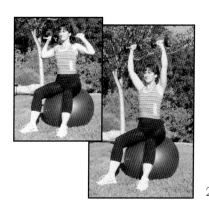

SHOULDER PRESS
(6 SLOW-MOTION REPS)

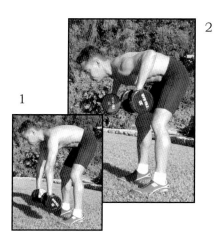

BENT OVER ROW
(6 SLOW-MOTION REPS)

BICEP CURL
(6 SLOW-MOTION REPS)

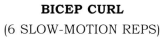
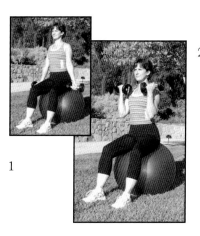

WEIGHT TRAINING FOR THE SIXTH FOURTEEN DAYS (15 minute session)

If you can, add some the weight to what you used in the last fourteen day segment. Complete one set of 6 reps of each exercise in slow motion (a slow count to 14 as you raise the weights and another slow count to 14 as you lower the weights). Remember to move from exercise to exercise as quickly as possible with no rest in between.

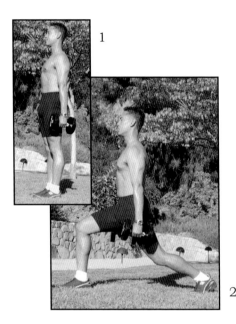

LUNGES
(6 SLOWMOTION REPS)

WALL SQUATS
(HOLD FOR 45-60 SECONDS)

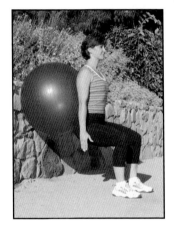

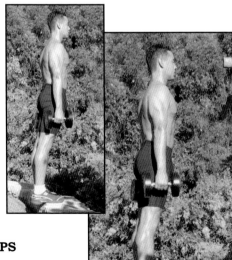

TOE UPS
(6 SLOW-MOTION
REPS)

YOGA/PILATES BLEND FOR THE SIXTH FOURTEEN DAYS
(15-20 minute session)

Flow from exercise to exercise doing the designated number of repetitions.

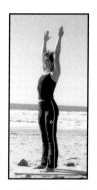

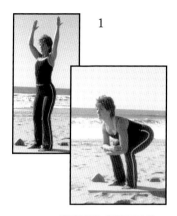

1

2

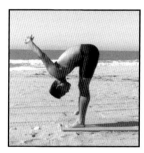

TALL MOUNTAIN

(3 BREATHS)

SUNFLOWERS

(5 BREATHS)

CHEST EXPANSION

(3 BREATHS)

PLANK

(1BREATH)

COBRA

(3 BREATHS)

DOWNWARD FACING
DOG

(3 BREATHS)

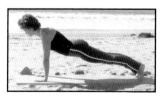 + 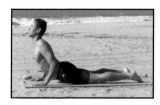 +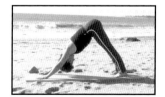

COMPLETE THE ABOVE SERIES (PLANK, COBRA, DOWN DOG)
THREE TIMES BEFORE MOVING ON TO SPINE STABILIZER.

YOGA/PILATES BLEND FOR THE SIXTH FOURTEEN DAYS
(15-20 minute session)

Flow from exercise to exercise doing the designated number of repetitions.

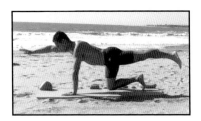

SPINE STABILIZER

(8 MOVEMENTS ALTERNATING SIDES)

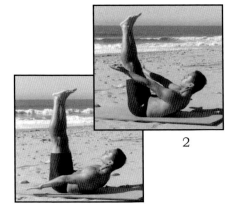

2

1

THE HUNDRED

(10 REPS)

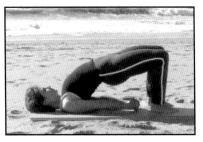

SHOULDER BRIDGE

(5 BREATHS)

2

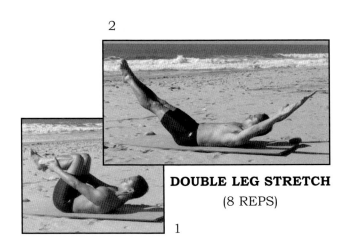

DOUBLE LEG STRETCH

(8 REPS)

1

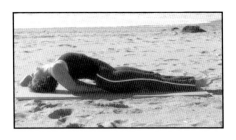

FISH POSE

(5 BREATHS)

YOGA/PILATES BLEND FOR THE SIXTH FOURTEEN DAYS
(15-20 minute session)

Flow from exercise to exercise doing the designated number of repetitions.

LEG CIRCLES
(8 REPS EACH LEG)

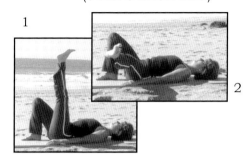

SPINE TWIST
(5 BREATHS)

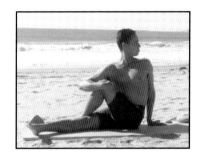

SIDE KICKS
(8 REPS EACH SIDE)

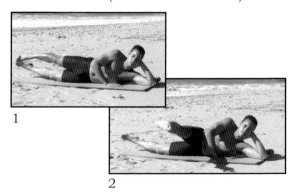

PIGEON POSE
(5 BREATHS)

Option A

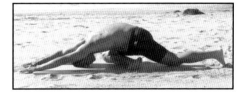

Option B

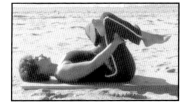

YOGA/PILATES BLEND FOR THE SIXTH FOURTEEN DAYS
(15-20 minute session)

Flow from exercise to exercise doing the designated number of repetitions.

SWIMMING
(8 BREATHS)

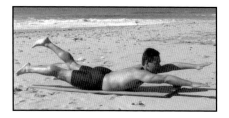

CHILD'S POSE
(5 BREATHS)

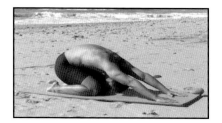

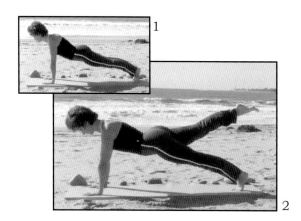

LEG PULL DOWNS
(8 REPS EACH SIDE)

CHILD'S POSE
(5 BREATHS)

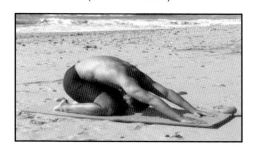

Day Seventy-one

☐   Fifteen minutes of meditation

☐   Cardio: Do thirty to forty-five minutes of alternating be-
      tween one minute of walking or jogging at a brisk pace,
      and walking or jogging at a moderate pace on a hilly
      course

☐   Weights: Do the suggested weight program with slow-
      motion repetitions for fifteen minutes moving from task to
      task with no rest in between

☐   Fifteen minutes of freeform journaling.

Whatever is worth
doing at all is
worth doing well.
-Phillip Stanhope

Notes for the day.....

_____

_____

_____

_____

_____

_____

Day Seventy-two

☐   Fifteen minutes of meditation

☐   Cardio: Do thirty to forty-five minutes of alternating be-
       tween one minute of walking or jogging at a brisk pace, and
       walking or jogging at a moderate pace on a hilly course

☐   Yoga/Pilates Blend: Do the suggested blend exercises for
       fifteen minutes with no rest in between

☐   Fifteen minutes of freeform journaling.

*I hold to the doc-
trine that with
ordinary talent, and
extraordinary
perseverence, all
things are attain-
able.
-Thomas Buxton*

Notes for the day.....

_____

_____

_____

_____

_____

_____

Day Seventy-three

☐ Fifteen minutes of meditation

☐ Cardio: Do thirty to forty-five minutes of alternating between one minute of walking or jogging at a brisk pace,
and walking or jogging at a moderate pace on a hilly
course

☐ Weights: Do the suggested weight program with slow-
motion repetitions for fifteen minutes moving from task to
task with no rest in between

☐ Fifteen minutes of freeform journaling.

Notes for the day.....

_____

_____

_____

_____

_____

_____

The aim of life is to live, and to live means to be awake, joyously, drunkenly, serenely, divinely aware.
-Henry Miller

Day Seventy-four

☐   Fifteen minutes of meditation

☐   Cardio: Do thirty to forty-five minutes of alternating between one minute of walking or jogging at a brisk pace, and walking or jogging at a moderate pace on a hilly course

☐   Yoga/Pilates Blend: Do the suggested blend exercises for fifteen minutes with no rest in between

☐   Fifteen minutes of freeform journaling.

A man travels the world over in search of what he needs and returns home to find it.
-George Moore

Notes for the day.....

_____

_____

_____

_____

_____

_____

Day Seventy-five

☐   Fifteen minutes of meditation

☐   Cardio: Do thirty to forty-five minutes of alternating between one minute of walking or jogging at a brisk pace,
and walking or jogging at a moderate pace on a hilly
course

☐   Weights: Do the suggested weight program with slow
motion repetitions for fifteen minutes moving from task to
task with no rest in between

☐   Fifteen minutes of freeform journaling.

Notes for the day.....

*Nothing great is
created suddenly
any more than a
bunch of grapes or
a fig.
-Epictetus*

_____

_____

_____

_____

_____

_____

Day Seventy-six

☐   Fifteen minutes of meditation

☐   Yoga/Pilates Blend: Do the suggested blend exercises for
     fifteen minutes with no rest in between

☐   Fifteen minutes of freeform journaling.

*Nothing splendid
has ever been
achieved except by
those who dared
believe that some-*   *Notes for the day.....*
*thing inside them
was superior to
circumstance.
-John Barton*

_____

_____

_____

_____

_____

_____

Day Seventy-seven

☐ Fifteen minutes of meditation

☐ This is a no exercise day and a cheat day for nutrition. Just try to eat healthy portions of foods that you love. Perhaps give yourself a special treat.

☐ Fifteen minutes of freeform journaling.

Notes for the day.....

Life's most urgent question is, what are you doing for others.
-Martin Luther King, Jr.

_____

_____

_____

_____

_____

_____

Day Seventy-eight

☐   Fifteen minutes of meditation

☐   Cardio: Do thirty to forty-five minutes of alternating between one minute of walking or jogging at a brisk pace, and
walking or jogging at a moderate pace on a hilly course

☐   Weights: Do the suggested weight program with slow-
motion repetitions for fifteen minutes moving from task to
task with no rest in between

☐   Fifteen minutes of freeform journaling.

*Great spirits have
always encoun-
tered violent
opposition from
mediocre minds.
-Albert Einstein*

Notes for the day.....

_____

_____

_____

_____

_____

_____

Day Seventy-nine

☐ Fifteen minutes of meditation

☐ Cardio: Do thirty to forty-five minutes of alternating between one minute of walking or jogging at a brisk pace, and walking or jogging at a moderate pace on a hilly course

☐ Yoga/Pilates Blend: Do the suggested blend exercises for fifteen minutes with no rest in between

☐ Fifteen minutes of freeform journaling.

Notes for the day.....

Neither a lofty degree of intelligence nor imagination nor both together go into the making of genius. Love, love, love. That is the soul of genius.
-Wolfgang Amadeus Mozart

_____

_____

_____

_____

_____

_____

Day Eighty

☐ Fifteen minutes of meditation

☐ Cardio: Do thirty to forty-five minutes of alternating between one minute of walking or jogging at a brisk pace, and walking or jogging at a moderate pace on a hilly course

☐ Weights: Do the suggested weight program with slow-motion repetitions for fifteen minutes moving from task to task with no rest in between

☐ Fifteen minutes of freeform journaling.

We cannot live only for ourselves. A thousand fibers connect us with our fellow-men; and along those fibers, as sympathetic threads, our actions run as causes, and they come back to us as effects.
-Herman Melville

Notes for the day.....

_____

_____

_____

_____

_____

_____

Day Eighty-one

☐ Fifteen minutes of meditation

☐ Cardio: Do thirty to forty-five minutes of alternating between one minute of walking or jogging at a brisk pace,
and walking or jogging at a moderate pace on a hilly
course

☐ Yoga/Pilates Blend: Do the suggested blend exercises for
fifteen minutes with no rest in between

☐ Fifteen minutes of freeform journaling.

Notes for the day.....

*Imagination is the
beginning of
creation. You
imagine what you
desire; you will
what you imagine,
and at last you
create what you
will.
-George Bernard
Shaw*

_____

_____

_____

_____

_____

_____

_____

Day Eighty-two

☐ Fifteen minutes of meditation

☐ Cardio: Do thirty to forty-five minutes of alternating between one minute of walking or jogging at a brisk pace, and walking or jogging at a moderate pace on a hilly course

☐ Weights: Do the suggested weight program with slow motion repetitions for fifteen minutes moving from task to task with no rest in between

☐ Fifteen minutes of freeform journaling.

A joyful heart is the inevitable result of a heart burning with love.
-Mother Teresa

Notes for the day.....

_____

_____

_____

_____

_____

_____

Day Eighty-three

☐   Fifteen minutes of meditation

☐   Yoga/Pilates Blend: Do the suggested blend exercises for fifteen minutes with no rest in between

☐   Fifteen minutes of freeform journaling.

Notes for the day.....

_____

_____

_____

_____

_____

_____

Many persons have a wrong idea of what constitutes true happiness. It is not attained through self-gratification, but through fidelity to a purpose.
-Helen Keller

Day Eighty-four

☐   Fifteen minutes of meditation

☐   This is a no exercise day and a cheat day for nutrition. Just
      try to eat healthy portions of foods that you love. Perhaps
      give yourself a special treat.

☐   Fifteen minutes of freeform journaling.

*Congratulations! You have completed the sixth two
weeks of Yin Yang Fitness.*

*Everything flows
on and on like
this river, without
pause, day and
night.
-Confucius*

Notes for the day.....

_____

_____

_____

_____

_____

_____

_____

You have completed the most difficult challenge—beginning.
You have created healthy changes and habits
that can stay within you for the rest of your life.
But only you can invite them to stay.